Introduction

Welcome to **"Plant-Based Fatty Liver Diet Cookbook: Nourishing Your Liver, One Plant-Based Meal at a Time."** If you're reading this, you may be seeking ways to improve your liver health and overall well-being through the power of plant-based nutrition. You've come to the right place.

Fatty liver disease, both alcoholic and non-alcoholic, is a growing concern for many people around the world. It can lead to serious health issues if left unmanaged, but the good news is that diet and lifestyle changes can have a profound impact on liver health. This cookbook is designed to provide you with delicious, nutritious, and easy-to-make recipes that support liver function and help you manage fatty liver disease effectively.

Why plant-based? Research has shown that a diet rich in plant-based foods can reduce liver fat, decrease inflammation, and improve liver function. By focusing on whole, unprocessed foods such as vegetables, fruits, whole grains, legumes, nuts, and seeds, you can give your liver the nutrients it needs to heal and thrive.

In this book, you'll find over 100 recipes that are not only liver-friendly but also packed with flavor. From hearty breakfasts and satisfying lunches to delicious dinners and delightful desserts, there's something here for every taste and occasion. Each recipe is crafted with ingredients known for their liver-supporting properties, making it easy for you to enjoy meals that are both healthful and enjoyable.

Beyond the recipes, this book also offers valuable information about fatty liver disease, including its causes, symptoms, and the science behind a plant-based diet's benefits. You'll also find practical tips for meal planning, grocery shopping, and maintaining a balanced diet that supports your liver health.

Whether you're new to plant-based eating or a seasoned pro, this cookbook will guide you on your journey to better liver health. Embrace the delicious, nourishing power of plants and take a proactive step toward a healthier, happier you. Let's start nourishing your liver, one plant-based meal at a time.

1. Roasted Brussels Sprouts with Balsamic Glaze

Ingredients:
- 1 1/2 lbs brussels sprouts, trimmed and halved
- 3 tbsp olive oil
- 1 tsp kosher salt
- 1/2 tsp black pepper
- 1/4 cup balsamic vinegar
- 2 tbsp brown sugar
- 2 tbsp butter

Instructions:

1. Preheat oven to 425°F. Line a baking sheet with foil or parchment paper.

2. In a large bowl, toss the brussels sprouts with the olive oil, salt and pepper until well coated. Spread out in a single layer on the prepared baking sheet.

3. Roast for 20-25 minutes, shaking the pan halfway, until sprouts are crisp-tender and browned.

4. While the sprouts roast, make the balsamic glaze. In a small saucepan, bring the balsamic vinegar and brown sugar to a simmer over medium heat. Allow to simmer for 5-7 minutes, stirring frequently, until mixture has reduced and thickened into a syrupy glaze.

5. Remove sprouts from oven and transfer to a serving bowl. Pour the balsamic glaze over the sprouts and toss to coat evenly. Add the butter and toss again until butter is melted and combined.

6. Serve the roasted brussels sprouts warm, garnished with extra balsamic glaze if desired.

The balsamic glaze adds a sweet, tangy contrast to the roasted, caramelized brussels sprouts. Enjoy!

2. Quinoa Vegetable Soup

Ingredients:
- 1 tbsp olive oil
- 1 onion, diced
- 3 carrots, peeled and sliced
- 3 celery stalks, sliced
- 4 cloves garlic, minced
- 6 cups vegetable or chicken broth
- 1 cup water
- 1 cup quinoa, rinsed
- 1 (15oz) can diced tomatoes
- 1 tsp dried basil
- 1 tsp dried oregano
- 1/2 tsp red pepper flakes (optional)
- Salt and pepper to taste
- 4 cups chopped kale or spinach
- Parmesan cheese for serving (optional)

Instructions:
1. In a large pot or dutch oven, heat the olive oil over medium-high heat. Add the onion, carrots and celery. Sauté for 5 minutes until vegetables are tender.

2. Add the garlic and cook for 1 minute more until fragrant.

3. Pour in the broth, water, quinoa, diced tomatoes, basil, oregano, red pepper flakes if using, and season with salt and pepper to taste.

4. Bring the soup to a boil, then reduce heat and simmer for 15-20 minutes, until quinoa is cooked through.

5. Stir in the chopped kale or spinach and cook for 2-3 minutes more until greens are wilted.

6. Taste and adjust seasonings as needed, adding more salt/pepper if desired.

7. Serve the quinoa vegetable soup warm, topped with grated parmesan cheese if you want.

This hearty vegetable soup is packed with protein from the quinoa and plenty of nutrients from all the veggies. It's a healthy, satisfying vegetarian meal. Adjust ingredients as needed for your taste preferences.

3. Kale and Sweet Potato Hash

Ingredients:
- 2 large sweet potatoes, peeled and diced into 1/2 inch cubes
- 2 tablespoons olive oil, divided
- 1 teaspoon smoked paprika
- 1/2 teaspoon ground cumin
- Salt and pepper to taste
- 1 bunch kale, stemmed and chopped (about 6 cups)
- 1 onion, diced
- 3 cloves garlic, minced
- 2 tablespoons apple cider vinegar
- 2 eggs (optional)

Instructions:
1. Preheat oven to 400°F. On a large baking sheet, toss the diced sweet potatoes with 1 tablespoon olive oil, smoked paprika, cumin, and a pinch each of salt and pepper. Spread in an even layer.

2. Roast for 20-25 minutes, flipping halfway, until sweet potatoes are fork-tender and browning.

3. Meanwhile, heat the remaining 1 tablespoon olive oil in a large skillet over medium heat. Add the onion and sauté for 5 minutes until translucent.

4. Add the garlic and chopped kale and continue cooking for 2-3 minutes, tossing frequently, until kale is wilted and garlic is fragrant.

5. Add the vinegar and season with salt and pepper to taste. Cook for 1 minute more.

6. Remove sweet potatoes from oven and add them to the skillet with the kale mixture. Toss everything together until well combined.

7. Optional: Create a well in the center of the hash and crack 2 eggs into it. Cover and cook until the eggs are done to your liking.

8. Serve the kale and sweet potato hash warm, either plain or topped with the cooked eggs if using.

This savory and nutritious hash makes a great breakfast, brunch or anytime meal. The roasted sweet potatoes add great flavor and texture contrasted by the wilted kale. Top with eggs for extra protein if desired.

4. Lentil and Vegetable Curry

Ingredients:
- 1 cup dried green or brown lentils, rinsed
- 1 tbsp olive oil
- 1 onion, diced
- 3 cloves garlic, minced
- 1 tbsp grated fresh ginger
- 1-2 tsp curry powder
- 1 tsp ground cumin
- 1 tsp ground coriander
- 1/2 tsp ground turmeric
- 1/4 tsp cayenne pepper (or to taste)
- 1 (14oz) can diced tomatoes
- 4 cups vegetable or chicken broth
- 1 sweet potato, peeled and diced
- 2 carrots, peeled and sliced
- 1 cup frozen peas
- Salt and pepper to taste
- Fresh cilantro for garnish
- Naan bread or cooked rice for serving

Instructions:
1. In a large pot, add the lentils and cover with water by 2 inches. Bring to a boil, then reduce heat and simmer for 15-20 minutes until lentils are tender but still hold their shape. Drain and set aside.

2. In the same pot, heat the olive oil over medium heat. Add the onion and sauté for 3-4 minutes until translucent.

3. Add the garlic, ginger, curry powder, cumin, coriander, turmeric and cayenne. Cook for 1 minute until fragrant.

4. Stir in the diced tomatoes with their juices and the vegetable broth. Add the cooked lentils, sweet potato, carrots and peas.

5. Season with salt and pepper to taste. Bring to a boil, then reduce heat and let simmer for 15-20 minutes until vegetables are fork-tender.

6. Taste and adjust seasonings as needed, adding more broth to thin the curry if desired.

7. Garnish with chopped fresh cilantro. Serve the lentil vegetable curry over basmati rice or with naan bread on the side.

This hearty, protein-packed lentil curry is loaded with vegetables and aromatic spices. It makes a satisfying vegan/vegetarian meal. You can adjust the heat level and vegetable mix to your tastes. Leftovers keep well too.

5. Grilled Portobello Mushroom Caps

Ingredients:
- 4 large portobello mushroom caps
- 1/4 cup olive oil
- 3 tablespoons balsamic vinegar
- 2 cloves garlic, minced
- 1 teaspoon dried basil
- 1 teaspoon dried oregano
- Salt and pepper to taste
- 4 slices provolone or mozzarella cheese (optional)

For Serving:
- Burger buns
- Lettuce, tomato, onion etc.

Instructions:

1. Clean the portobello caps by wiping with a damp paper towel to remove any dirt/debris. Gently twist off the stems.

2. In a shallow baking dish, whisk together the olive oil, balsamic vinegar, garlic, dried basil, oregano, salt and pepper.

3. Add the portobello caps to the dish and use a spoon to coat them evenly with the marinade on both sides. Let marinate for 30 minutes at room temperature.

4. Pre-heat grill to medium-high heat and lightly oil the grates.

5. Remove portobellos from marinade and place cap-side down on the hot grill grates. Grill for 5 minutes until grill marks appear.

6. Flip over and grill for 3-5 minutes more until mushrooms are tender.

7. If adding cheese, place a slice on each cap during the last 2 minutes of grilling to allow it to melt.

8. Remove grilled portobellos from heat and let rest for 5 minutes.

9. Toast burger buns if desired and assemble the mushroom caps with your favorite toppings like lettuce, tomato, onion etc.

These balsamic marinated grilled portobello caps make a delicious vegetarian burger option. The mushrooms get tender and meaty with a savory punch of flavor from the marinade. You can enjoy them plain or dress them up like a burger on a bun.

6. Baked Tofu with Stir-Fried Veggies

Ingredients:
- 1 (14oz) block extra-firm tofu, drained and cut into 1-inch cubes
- 2 tbsp soy sauce or tamari
- 1 tbsp rice vinegar
- 1 tbsp toasted sesame oil
- 1 tsp garlic powder
- 1/4 tsp ground ginger

Stir-Fried Veggies:
- 2 tbsp vegetable or peanut oil
- 1 bell pepper, sliced
- 1 cup broccoli florets
- 1 cup sliced mushrooms
- 1 cup snow peas
- 3 cloves garlic, minced
- 1 tsp sesame seeds
- Salt and pepper to taste

Instructions:
1. Preheat oven to 400°F. Line a baking sheet with parchment paper or foil.

2. In a shallow bowl, whisk together the soy sauce, rice vinegar, sesame oil, garlic powder and ginger. Add the cubed tofu and gently toss to coat. Let marinate for 10-15 minutes.

3. Arrange the marinated tofu in an even layer on the prepared baking sheet. Bake for 20 minutes, flipping halfway, until lightly browned.

4. While the tofu bakes, prepare the veggies. Heat the oil in a large skillet or wok over high heat. Add the bell pepper, broccoli, mushrooms and snow peas. Stir-fry for 4-5 minutes until crisp-tender.

5. Add the minced garlic and sesame seeds and toss for 30 seconds until fragrant. Season with salt and pepper to taste.

6. Once tofu is baked, add it to the veggie stir-fry and gently toss everything together.

7. Serve the baked tofu and stir-fried veggies over rice or noodles if desired. Garnish with extra sesame seeds and sliced green onions.

This baked tofu has amazing texture and flavor from the marinade. Paired with the fresh stir-fried veggies, it makes a healthy, plant-based meal that is satisfying and delicious.

7. Cauliflower Rice Stir-Fry

Ingredients:
- 1 large head cauliflower, riced (or 4 cups cauliflower rice)
- 2 tbsp sesame oil
- 1 cup frozen peas and carrots, thawed
- 1 bell pepper, diced
- 4 oz mushrooms, sliced
- 3 cloves garlic, minced
- 2 eggs, beaten
- 3 tbsp low-sodium soy sauce
- 2 tsp rice vinegar
- 1 tsp ground ginger
- 2 green onions, sliced
- Salt and pepper to taste

Instructions:

1. If using a head of cauliflower, rice it using a box grater or pulse in a food processor until it resembles rice-sized granules.

2. Heat 1 tbsp of the sesame oil in a large skillet or wok over medium-high heat. Add the riced cauliflower and stir-fry for 2-3 minutes until tender-crisp. Transfer to a plate.

3. Return skillet to heat and add remaining 1 tbsp sesame oil. Add the peas, carrots, bell pepper and mushrooms. Stir-fry for 3-4 minutes.

4. Push veggies to the sides and crack the eggs into the center of the skillet. Scramble the eggs, breaking them up into smaller pieces with a spatula as they cook.

5. Once eggs are cooked through, mix them together with the veggies. Add the cauliflower rice back in.

6. Whisk together the soy sauce, rice vinegar and ginger. Pour over the stir-fry and toss everything to combine and coat evenly.

7. Allow to cook for 2 more minutes, stirring frequently, to heat through and let flavors meld. Remove from heat and stir in the sliced green onions. Season with salt and pepper to taste.

This veggie-packed cauliflower rice stir-fry is a low-carb, nutrient dense meal. You get all the flavors of traditional fried rice but using riced cauliflower as the base. Quick, easy and versatile - add any other veggies you like!

8. Veggie-Packed Chili

Ingredients:
- 1 tbsp olive oil
- 1 onion, diced
- 3 cloves garlic, minced
- 2 carrots, peeled and diced
- 2 bell peppers, diced
- 2 zucchini, diced
- 1 (14oz) can diced tomatoes
- 1 (15oz) can tomato sauce
- 1 (15oz) can kidney beans, drained and rinsed
- 1 (15oz) can black beans, drained and rinsed
- 2 cups vegetable broth
- 2 tbsp chili powder
- 1 tsp ground cumin
- 1 tsp smoked paprika
- 1 tsp oregano
- 1/2 tsp cayenne (or to taste)
- Salt and pepper to taste
- Diced avocado, shredded cheese, sour cream for serving (optional)

Instructions:

1. In a large pot or dutch oven, heat the olive oil over medium-high heat. Add the diced onion and sauté for 3-4 minutes until translucent.

2. Add the garlic, carrots, bell peppers and zucchini. Cook for 5 minutes, stirring frequently, until veggies are tender-crisp.

3. Pour in the diced tomatoes with juices, tomato sauce, drained beans, vegetable broth, chili powder, cumin, smoked paprika, oregano and cayenne.

4. Season with salt and pepper to taste. Bring to a simmer and let the chili cook for 20-25 minutes to allow the flavors to develop.

5. Taste and adjust seasoning if needed, adding more spices, salt/pepper etc. If too thick, add a splash more veggie broth.

6. Let chili continue simmering for 10-15 more minutes until thickened to your desired consistency.

7. Serve the veggie chili hot, garnished with diced avocado, shredded cheese, sour cream or any other desired toppings.

This veggie-packed chili is hearty, filling, and loaded with nutrients from all the different vegetables and beans. It's a warm, comforting meal that is vegetarian/vegan-friendly and easy to customize to your tastes.

9. Roasted Beet and Arugula Salad

Ingredients:
- 4-5 medium beets, greens removed
- 2 tbsp olive oil
- 1 tsp balsamic vinegar
- Salt and pepper
- 5 oz arugula
- 1/2 cup toasted walnuts
- 1/3 cup crumbled goat or feta cheese
- 2 tbsp balsamic vinaigrette

For the Balsamic Vinaigrette:
- 1/4 cup olive oil
- 2 tbsp balsamic vinegar
- 1 tsp dijon mustard
- 1 garlic clove, minced
- Salt and pepper to taste

Instructions:
1. Preheat oven to 400°F. Scrub the beets and trim any stems/roots. Toss with 2 tbsp olive oil, 1 tsp balsamic vinegar, and salt and pepper.

2. Wrap the beets individually in foil packets and place on a baking sheet. Roast for 50-60 minutes until fork tender.

3. Meanwhile, make the vinaigrette by whisking together the olive oil, balsamic vinegar, mustard, garlic and salt and pepper.

4. Once beets are cool enough to handle, peel them and cut into wedges or chunks.

5. In a large bowl, toss the roasted beet pieces with the arugula, walnuts, and cheese.

6. Drizzle the balsamic vinaigrette over top and toss gently to coat everything evenly.

7. Serve the beet and arugula salad immediately while the beets are still slightly warm. Add extra cracked pepper on top if desired.

The roasted beets give this salad a delicious sweet and earthy flavor that pairs perfectly with the peppery arugula, creamy cheese, and tangy balsamic vinaigrette. Toasted walnuts add a great crunch. You can prepare the ingredients ahead of time for easy assembly.

10. Stuffed Bell Peppers with Quinoa

Ingredients:
- 6 bell peppers, tops cut off and seeds/membranes removed
- 1 cup quinoa, rinsed
- 2 cups vegetable or chicken broth
- 1 tbsp olive oil
- 1 onion, diced
- 2 cloves garlic, minced
- 1 cup cooked black beans or lentils
- 1 cup frozen corn kernels
- 1 cup diced tomatoes
- 1 tsp cumin
- 1 tsp chili powder
- 1/2 tsp smoked paprika
- Salt and pepper to taste
- 1 cup shredded cheese (Mexican, cheddar, etc)
- Fresh cilantro for garnish

Instructions:

1. Preheat oven to 375°F. Cook the quinoa by combining it with the broth in a saucepan. Bring to a boil, then reduce heat and simmer covered for 15-20 minutes until liquid is absorbed. Fluff with a fork.

2. Meanwhile, heat the olive oil in a skillet over medium heat. Sauté the onion for 3-4 minutes until translucent. Add the garlic and cook 1 minute more until fragrant.

3. Add the cooked black beans or lentils, frozen corn, diced tomatoes, cumin, chili powder, smoked paprika and salt and pepper to taste. Stir to combine.

4. Remove from heat and stir in the cooked quinoa until fully incorporated.

5. Stuff the hollowed out bell pepper halves evenly with the quinoa filling, packing it down gently.

6. Place the stuffed peppers upright in a baking dish. Pour a small amount of broth or water into the bottom of the dish.

7. Cover with foil and bake for 30 minutes. Remove foil, top with shredded cheese and bake uncovered 10-15 more minutes until cheese is melted.

8. Serve the stuffed bell peppers warm, garnished with fresh chopped cilantro if desired.

These hearty vegetarian stuffed peppers are nutrient-dense and full of southwestern flavors. Quinoa makes a protein-packed filling along with beans, veggies and spices. Customize with your favorite fillings!

11. Vegetable Frittata

Ingredients:
- 8 large eggs
- 1/4 cup milk or unsweetened non-dairy milk
- 1/2 tsp salt
- 1/4 tsp black pepper
- 1 tbsp olive oil or butter
- 1/2 onion, diced
- 1 cup sliced mushrooms
- 1 cup broccoli florets, chopped into small pieces
- 1 bell pepper, diced
- 2 cloves garlic, minced
- 1 cup baby spinach
- 1/2 cup shredded cheddar, feta, or your favorite cheese

Instructions:

1. Preheat oven to 350°F. Grease a 9-inch pie pan or oven-safe skillet with butter or non-stick cooking spray.

2. In a large bowl, whisk together the eggs, milk, salt and pepper until fully combined. Set aside.

3. Heat the olive oil or butter in a skillet over medium heat. Add the onions and sauté for 2 minutes until translucent.

4. Add the mushrooms, broccoli, bell pepper and garlic. Continue sautéing for 5 minutes until vegetables are tender.

5. Add the baby spinach and cook for 1 minute more until it wilts down. Remove from heat.

6. Spread the sautéed vegetables evenly in the prepared pie pan or skillet. Pour the egg mixture over top.

7. Use a fork to gently lift the vegetables up and allow the eggs to spread evenly over the bottom.

8. Sprinkle the shredded cheese evenly over top.

9. Bake for 20-25 minutes until the center is set and the top is lightly golden brown.

10. Allow the frittata to cool for 5 minutes before slicing into wedges and serving warm.

This veggie-packed frittata is a delicious protein-rich breakfast or brunch dish. You can customize it with your choice of vegetables, cheeses, and fresh herbs. Easily made ahead for quick reheating too!

12. Sweet Potato and Black Bean Burrito Bowls

Ingredients:
- 2 large sweet potatoes, peeled and diced into 1/2-inch cubes
- 2 tbsp olive oil, divided
- 1 tsp chili powder
- 1 tsp cumin
- 1/2 tsp smoked paprika
- Salt and pepper to taste
- 1 (14oz) can black beans, drained and rinsed
- 1 cup cooked brown rice
- 1 cup frozen corn kernels
- 1 avocado, diced
- 2 roma tomatoes, diced
- 1/4 red onion, diced
- 1 lime, cut into wedges
- Chopped cilantro for garnish
- Hot sauce or salsa for serving (optional)

Instructions:

1. Preheat oven to 400°F. Toss the diced sweet potatoes with 1 tbsp olive oil, chili powder, cumin, smoked paprika and salt and pepper on a baking sheet. Roast for 20-25 minutes until tender.

2. In a skillet, heat the remaining 1 tbsp olive oil over medium heat. Add the drained black beans and warm through, smashing some with a fork to create a rough mash.

3. Prepare the brown rice according to package instructions.

4. To assemble the burrito bowls, divide the roasted sweet potatoes, black bean mash, brown rice, frozen corn, avocado, tomatoes and red onion between 4 bowls.

5. Squeeze a lime wedge over each bowl and garnish with chopped cilantro.

6. Serve the burrito bowls warm, with hot sauce or salsa for adding extra kick if desired.

These hearty vegetarian burrito bowls are packed with plant-based protein and fiber from the sweet potatoes, black beans and brown rice. You get lots of fresh flavors and textures from the tomatoes, avocado, corn and lime. Easily customizable with your favorite toppings!

13. Mediterranean Chickpea Salad

Ingredients:
- 1 (15oz) can chickpeas, drained and rinsed
- 1 cucumber, diced
- 1 red bell pepper, diced
- 1/2 red onion, diced
- 1 cup cherry tomatoes, halved
- 1/2 cup pitted kalamata olives
- 1/2 cup crumbled feta cheese
- 1/4 cup chopped fresh parsley
- 1/4 cup chopped fresh mint

For the Dressing:
- 1/4 cup olive oil
- 3 tbsp red wine vinegar
- 1 tbsp lemon juice
- 2 cloves garlic, minced
- 1 tsp dried oregano
- 1/2 tsp Dijon mustard
- Salt and pepper to taste

Instructions:
1. In a large bowl, combine the chickpeas, diced cucumber, bell pepper, red onion, cherry tomatoes, olives and feta.

2. Add the chopped fresh parsley and mint.

3. In a small bowl or jar, whisk together the olive oil, red wine vinegar, lemon juice, garlic, oregano, Dijon and salt and pepper.

4. Pour the dressing over the chickpea salad and toss gently to combine.

5. Let the salad marinate for 15-30 minutes to allow flavors to meld.

6. Give it one more gentle toss before serving to re-distribute the dressing.

7. Garnish with extra parsley and feta if desired. Serve chilled or at room temperature.

This bright and fresh Mediterranean chickpea salad is loaded with plant-based protein and fiber. The mix of fresh veggies, briny olives and feta along with the zesty dressing packs so much flavor. It's perfect for meal prep, easy lunches or as a side salad.

14. Grilled Eggplant with Tomato Salsa

Ingredients:

For the Grilled Eggplant:
- 2 medium eggplants, sliced into 1/2-inch rounds
- 2 tbsp olive oil
- Salt and pepper to taste

For the Tomato Salsa:
- 2 cups diced tomatoes
- 1/2 cup diced red onion
- 2 cloves garlic, minced
- 1 jalapeño, seeded and minced (optional for heat)
- 1/4 cup chopped fresh cilantro
- 2 tbsp lime juice
- Salt and pepper to taste

Instructions:

1. Preheat grill or grill pan to medium-high heat. Brush the eggplant rounds with olive oil on both sides and season with salt and pepper.

2. Grill the eggplant for 4-5 minutes per side, until tender and char marks appear. Transfer to a plate when done.

3. To make the salsa: In a bowl, mix together the diced tomatoes, red onion, garlic, jalapeño (if using), cilantro, lime juice, and salt and pepper to taste.

4. Let the salsa sit for 10-15 minutes to allow flavors to blend.

5. To serve, arrange the grilled eggplant rounds on a platter and top each slice generously with the fresh tomato salsa.

6. Optionally, you can drizzle with extra virgin olive oil or add crumbled feta or queso fresco on top.

The smoky grilled eggplant pairs perfectly with the bright, zesty tomato salsa in this vegetarian dish. It makes a wonderful appetizer, light main course or tasty side. The salsa can be made a few hours in advance to allow flavors to develop further.

15. Lentil and Vegetable Shepherd's Pie

Ingredients:
- 1 cup dried green or brown lentils, rinsed

For the Mashed Potato Topping:
- 2 lbs potatoes, peeled and cut into chunks
- 1/2 cup milk or unsweetened non-dairy milk
- 2 tbsp butter or olive oil
- Salt and pepper to taste

- 2 cups vegetable or mushroom broth
- 2 tbsp olive oil
- 1 onion, diced
- 2 carrots, peeled and diced
- 2 celery stalks, diced
- 8 oz mushrooms, sliced
- 2 cloves garlic, minced
- 1 tsp dried thyme
- 1 tsp tomato paste
- 1 cup frozen peas
- Salt and pepper to taste

Instructions:

1. In a saucepan, combine the lentils and broth. Bring to a boil, then reduce heat and simmer for 15-20 minutes until lentils are tender but still hold their shape.

2. Preheat oven to 400°F. Grease a 9x13 baking dish.

3. Heat the olive oil in a skillet over medium-high heat. Sauté the onions, carrots, celery, and mushrooms for 5-7 minutes until softened.

4. Add the garlic, thyme, and tomato paste. Cook for 1 minute until fragrant.

5. Add the cooked lentils along with any remaining cooking liquid to the skillet. Stir in the frozen peas and season with salt and pepper to taste.

6. Transfer the lentil vegetable mixture to the prepared baking dish and spread evenly.

7. Meanwhile, make the mashed potato topping: Boil the potato chunks until fork tender, then drain.

8. Mash the potatoes with the milk/non-dairy milk and butter/olive oil until smooth. Season with salt and pepper.

9. Spread the mashed potatoes evenly over the top of the lentil filling. Bake for 20-25 minutes until heated through and lightly browned on top. Let cool for 5-10 minutes before serving hot.

This veggie and lentil shepherd's pie is a fantastic meatless take on the classic comfort food. It's hearty, savory, and loaded with nutritious lentils, mushrooms and vegetables under a creamy mashed potato topping.

16. Vegetable Fried Rice

Ingredients:
- 3 cups cooked and cooled rice (day-old is best)
- 2 tbsp sesame oil
- 1 cup frozen mixed vegetables (carrots, peas, corn), thawed
- 1/2 cup finely diced onion
- 2 cloves garlic, minced
- 2 eggs, lightly beaten
- 2 green onions, sliced
- 3 tbsp low-sodium soy sauce
- 1 tsp rice vinegar (optional)
- Salt and pepper to taste

Instructions:

1. If using freshly cooked rice, spread it out on a baking sheet to cool completely before using for fried rice.

2. Heat 1/2 tbsp of the sesame oil in a large skillet or wok over medium-high heat. Pour in the beaten eggs and swirl to coat the pan. Cook, pushing the eggs around, until scrambled and set. Remove eggs to a plate.

3. Add the remaining 1 1/2 tbsp sesame oil to the wok. Add the frozen mixed veggies, onion and garlic. Stir-fry for 2 minutes.

4. Add the cooled rice and use a spatula or spoon to break it apart and toss with the veggie mixture.

5. Drizzle the soy sauce over top and toss to incorporate. Let the rice cook for 2-3 minutes to get heated through, stirring frequently.

6. Add the scrambled eggs back in and toss to combine with the rice.

7. Remove from heat and stir in the green onions and rice vinegar (if using). Season with salt and pepper to taste.

8. Serve the vegetable fried rice immediately while hot.

This is a great vegetarian version of classic fried rice loaded up with a mix of healthy veggies and scrambled egg. Using cooled, day-old rice helps prevent the fried rice from getting mushy. Feel free to add in any other diced veggies you'd like.

17. Roasted Broccoli with Garlic

Ingredients:
- 1 large head of broccoli, cut into florets
- 4 cloves of garlic, minced
- 2 tablespoons olive oil
- Salt and pepper to taste
- Optional: Parmesan cheese for topping

Instructions:

1. Preheat your oven to 425°F (220°C).

2. In a large bowl, toss the broccoli florets with minced garlic, olive oil, salt, and pepper until the broccoli is evenly coated.

3. Spread the broccoli out in a single layer on a baking sheet lined with parchment paper or aluminum foil. Make sure the florets are not overcrowded to ensure even roasting.

4. Roast the broccoli in the preheated oven for 20-25 minutes, or until the edges are crispy and the broccoli is tender when pierced with a fork. You may want to flip the broccoli halfway through cooking for even browning.

5. Once roasted, remove the broccoli from the oven and transfer it to a serving dish. If desired, sprinkle freshly grated Parmesan cheese over the top before serving.

6. Enjoy your roasted broccoli with garlic as a tasty side dish alongside your favorite main course!

Feel free to adjust the seasoning according to your taste preferences, and you can also add other spices or herbs like red pepper flakes or thyme for extra flavor.

18. Vegetarian Sushi Rolls

Ingredients:
- 2 cups sushi rice
- 4 cups water
- 1/2 cup rice vinegar
- 2 tablespoons sugar
- Nori sheets (seaweed)
- 1 teaspoon salt
- Assorted vegetables for filling (such as cucumber, avocado, carrot, bell pepper, asparagus, and/or tofu)
- Soy sauce, pickled ginger, and wasabi for serving

Instructions:

1. Rinse the sushi rice under cold water until the water runs clear. Drain well.

2. In a rice cooker or medium saucepan, combine the rinsed rice and water. Cook the rice according to the package instructions.

3. While the rice is cooking, prepare the sushi vinegar. In a small saucepan, combine the rice vinegar, sugar, and salt. Heat over low heat until the sugar and salt dissolve. Remove from heat and let it cool.

4. Once the rice is cooked, transfer it to a large bowl and let it cool slightly. While it's still warm, gently fold in the sushi vinegar mixture until well combined. Be careful not to mash the rice.

5. Prepare your filling ingredients by slicing them into thin strips or julienne.

6. Place a sheet of nori on a bamboo sushi rolling mat or a clean kitchen towel.

7. Wet your hands lightly with water to prevent sticking, then spread a thin layer of sushi rice evenly over the nori, leaving about 1 inch of the nori sheet uncovered at the top.

8. Arrange your desired fillings in a line across the center of the rice.

9. Using the sushi mat or towel, tightly roll up the sushi, starting from the bottom edge, pressing gently to seal.

10. Repeat the process with the remaining nori sheets and filling ingredients.

11. Once all the rolls are assembled, use a sharp knife to slice each roll into individual pieces, wiping the knife with a damp cloth between cuts to keep it clean.

12. Serve the vegetarian sushi rolls with soy sauce, pickled ginger, and wasabi on the side.

13. Enjoy your homemade vegetarian sushi rolls as a delicious and healthy meal or snack!

19. Butternut Squash Soup

Ingredients:
- 1 medium butternut squash (about 2 pounds), peeled, seeded, and cut into 1-inch cubes
- 1 onion, chopped
- 2 carrots, chopped
- 2 celery stalks, chopped
- 3 cloves garlic, minced
- 4 cups vegetable broth
- 1 teaspoon dried thyme
- 1/2 teaspoon ground cinnamon
- 1/4 teaspoon ground nutmeg
- Salt and pepper to taste
- 2 tablespoons olive oil
- Optional toppings: roasted pumpkin seeds, croutons, sour cream, or fresh herbs

Instructions:

1. Heat the olive oil in a large pot over medium heat. Add the chopped onion, carrots, and celery. Cook, stirring occasionally, until the vegetables are softened, about 5-7 minutes.

2. Add the minced garlic to the pot and cook for an additional 1-2 minutes, until fragrant.

3. Add the cubed butternut squash to the pot, along with the vegetable broth, dried thyme, ground cinnamon, and ground nutmeg. Stir to combine.

4. Bring the soup to a boil, then reduce the heat to low and simmer, covered, for about 20-25 minutes, or until the butternut squash is tender.

5. Once the squash is cooked, remove the pot from the heat. Use an immersion blender to puree the soup until smooth and creamy. Alternatively, you can carefully transfer the soup in batches to a blender and blend until smooth, then return it to the pot.

6. Season the soup with salt and pepper to taste, adjusting as needed.

7. If the soup is too thick, you can add more vegetable broth or water to reach your desired consistency.

8. Serve the butternut squash soup hot, garnished with your choice of toppings such as roasted pumpkin seeds, croutons, a dollop of sour cream, or fresh herbs. Enjoy the warm and comforting flavors of homemade butternut squash soup!

This soup can be easily customized to suit your taste preferences. You can add a splash of coconut milk for extra creaminess or a pinch of cayenne pepper for a hint of heat. Feel free to experiment with different spices and toppings to make it your own!

20. Quinoa and Black Bean Stuffed Tomatoes

Ingredients:
- 4 large tomatoes
- 1 cup cooked quinoa
- 1 can (15 ounces) black beans, drained and rinsed
- 1 bell pepper, diced
- 1/2 red onion, diced
- 2 cloves garlic, minced
- 1 teaspoon ground cumin
- 1/2 teaspoon chili powder
- Salt and pepper to taste
- 1/4 cup chopped fresh cilantro or parsley
- 1 cup shredded cheese (such as cheddar or Monterey Jack), optional

Instructions:

1. Preheat your oven to 375°F (190°C).

2. Slice off the tops of the tomatoes and carefully scoop out the seeds and pulp using a spoon, leaving a hollow cavity. Set the hollowed-out tomatoes aside.

3. In a large mixing bowl, combine the cooked quinoa, black beans, diced bell pepper, diced red onion, minced garlic, ground cumin, chili powder, salt, pepper, and chopped cilantro or parsley. Mix well to combine.

4. Spoon the quinoa and black bean mixture into the hollowed-out tomatoes, pressing down gently to pack the filling.

5. If using cheese, sprinkle it over the top of each stuffed tomato.

6. Place the stuffed tomatoes in a baking dish or on a baking sheet lined with parchment paper.

7. Bake in the preheated oven for 20-25 minutes, or until the tomatoes are tender and the filling is heated through.

8. Once baked, remove the stuffed tomatoes from the oven and let them cool slightly before serving.

9. Serve the quinoa and black bean stuffed tomatoes garnished with additional chopped cilantro or parsley, if desired.

10. Enjoy your delicious and wholesome quinoa and black bean stuffed tomatoes!

These stuffed tomatoes are versatile, so feel free to customize the filling with your favorite ingredients, such as corn, diced avocado, or jalapeños. They also make a great meal prep option and can be enjoyed warm or cold.

21. Kale and Edamame Salad

Ingredients:
- 4 cups chopped kale leaves, tough stems removed
- 1 cup cooked and shelled edamame (thawed if using frozen)
- 1/2 cup grated carrots
- 1/4 cup sliced red onion
- 1/4 cup sliced almonds or roasted sunflower seeds
- 1/4 cup dried cranberries or raisins
- Optional: crumbled feta cheese or grated Parmesan cheese

For the dressing:
- 3 tablespoons olive oil
- 2 tablespoons lemon juice (about 1 lemon)
- 1 tablespoon Dijon mustard
- 1 garlic clove, minced
- Salt and pepper to taste

Instructions:
1. In a small bowl, whisk together the olive oil, lemon juice, Dijon mustard, minced garlic, salt, and pepper to make the dressing. Set aside.

2. In a large mixing bowl, add the chopped kale leaves. Pour half of the dressing over the kale and massage it with your hands for a few minutes until the kale begins to soften and wilt slightly.

3. Add the cooked edamame, grated carrots, sliced red onion, sliced almonds or sunflower seeds, and dried cranberries or raisins to the bowl with the kale.

4. Pour the remaining dressing over the salad and toss everything together until well combined.

5. If using, sprinkle crumbled feta cheese or grated Parmesan cheese over the top of the salad.

6. Taste and adjust the seasoning, adding more salt and pepper if needed. Serve the kale and edamame salad immediately as a nutritious side dish or light meal. Enjoy the vibrant flavors and textures of this delicious salad!

This salad can be easily customized based on your preferences. Feel free to add other vegetables, nuts, or seeds, and adjust the dressing ingredients to suit your taste. It also makes a great option for meal prep and can be stored in the refrigerator for a few days, allowing the flavors to meld together even more.

22. Zucchini Noodles with Pesto

Ingredients:
- 4 medium zucchinis
- 1 cup fresh basil leaves
- 1/4 cup pine nuts or walnuts
- 2 cloves garlic
- 1/4 cup grated Parmesan cheese (optional)
- 1/4 cup extra virgin olive oil
- Salt and pepper to taste
- Optional toppings: cherry tomatoes, sliced olives, grilled chicken, or shrimp

Instructions:

1. Using a spiralizer or a julienne peeler, create zucchini noodles (also known as zoodles) by shredding the zucchinis into long, thin strands. Alternatively, you can use a sharp knife to slice the zucchinis thinly into noodle-like strips.

2. Place the zucchini noodles in a colander set over a bowl and sprinkle them with a pinch of salt. Toss to combine and let them sit for about 10-15 minutes to allow excess moisture to drain.

3. Meanwhile, prepare the pesto sauce. In a food processor or blender, combine the fresh basil leaves, pine nuts or walnuts, garlic cloves, and grated Parmesan cheese (if using). Pulse until the ingredients are finely chopped.

4. With the food processor running, slowly drizzle in the olive oil until the pesto reaches your desired consistency. You may need to stop and scrape down the sides of the bowl with a spatula.

5. Season the pesto with salt and pepper to taste, adjusting as needed.

6. Once the zucchini noodles have drained, gently squeeze them with your hands to remove any remaining moisture.

7. Heat a large skillet over medium heat and add a drizzle of olive oil. Add the zucchini noodles to the skillet and sauté for 2-3 minutes, or until they are just tender but still have a slight crunch.

8. Add the pesto sauce to the skillet with the zucchini noodles and toss to coat evenly. Cook for an additional minute, stirring occasionally, until the pesto is heated through.

9. Remove the skillet from the heat and serve the zucchini noodles with pesto immediately, topped with your choice of optional toppings such as cherry tomatoes, sliced olives, grilled chicken, or shrimp.

10. Enjoy your light and flavorful zucchini noodles with pesto as a satisfying and healthy meal!

23. Roasted Brussels Sprouts and Sweet Potato Hash

Ingredients:
- 2 cups Brussels sprouts, trimmed and halved
- 2 medium sweet potatoes, peeled and diced into small cubes
- 1 onion, chopped
- 2 cloves garlic, minced
- 2 tablespoons olive oil
- 1 teaspoon smoked paprika
- 1/2 teaspoon dried thyme
- Salt and pepper to taste
- Optional toppings: fried or poached eggs, avocado slices, chopped fresh herbs

Instructions:

1. Preheat your oven to 425°F (220°C).

2. In a large mixing bowl, toss the halved Brussels sprouts, diced sweet potatoes, chopped onion, and minced garlic with olive oil until well coated.

3. Spread the mixture out in a single layer on a baking sheet lined with parchment paper or aluminum foil.

4. Sprinkle the smoked paprika, dried thyme, salt, and pepper over the vegetables, tossing gently to evenly distribute the seasonings.

5. Roast the Brussels sprouts and sweet potatoes in the preheated oven for 20-25 minutes, or until the vegetables are tender and caramelized, stirring halfway through cooking.

6. Once roasted, remove the baking sheet from the oven and transfer the roasted Brussels sprouts and sweet potatoes to a serving dish.

7. Serve the hash hot, topped with your choice of optional toppings such as fried or poached eggs, avocado slices, or chopped fresh herbs.

8. Enjoy the delicious combination of flavors and textures in this roasted Brussels sprouts and sweet potato hash!

Feel free to customize this dish by adding other vegetables such as bell peppers, mushrooms, or kale. You can also adjust the seasonings to your taste preferences, adding more smoked paprika for extra smokiness or a sprinkle of red pepper flakes for a hint of heat. This versatile hash makes a satisfying and nutritious meal any time of day.

24. Lentil Sloppy Joes

Ingredients:
- 1 cup dry green or brown lentils
- 2 1/2 cups vegetable broth or water
- 1 tablespoon olive oil
- 1 onion, finely chopped
- 2 cloves garlic, minced
- 1 bell pepper, diced
- 1 carrot, grated
- 1 can (15 ounces) tomato sauce
- 2 tablespoons tomato paste
- 2 tablespoons maple syrup or brown sugar
- 1 tablespoon Worcestershire sauce (use vegan if desired)
- 1 tablespoon apple cider vinegar
- 1 teaspoon chili powder
- 1/2 teaspoon ground cumin
- Salt and pepper to taste
- Hamburger buns or bread rolls, for serving

Instructions:
1. Rinse the lentils under cold water and drain.

2. In a medium saucepan, combine the lentils and vegetable broth or water. Bring to a boil, then reduce the heat to low and simmer, covered, for about 20-25 minutes, or until the lentils are tender but not mushy. Drain any excess liquid and set the lentils aside.

3. In a large skillet, heat the olive oil over medium heat. Add the chopped onion, minced garlic, diced bell pepper, and grated carrot. Cook, stirring occasionally, for about 5-7 minutes, or until the vegetables are softened.

4. Add the cooked lentils to the skillet with the sautéed vegetables.

5. In a small bowl, whisk together the tomato sauce, tomato paste, maple syrup or brown sugar, Worcestershire sauce, apple cider vinegar, chili powder, ground cumin, salt, and pepper.

6. Pour the sauce mixture over the lentils and vegetables in the skillet. Stir to combine.

7. Reduce the heat to low and simmer the lentil mixture for about 10-15 minutes, stirring occasionally, to allow the flavors to meld together and the sauce to thicken.

8. Taste and adjust the seasoning, adding more salt and pepper if needed. Once the lentil mixture has thickened to your desired consistency, remove the skillet from the heat.

9. To serve, spoon the lentil sloppy joe mixture onto hamburger buns or bread rolls. Enjoy your delicious and hearty lentil sloppy joes!

Feel free to customize your lentil sloppy joes by adding your favorite toppings such as sliced pickles, shredded lettuce, or sliced onions. This plant-based version of a classic comfort food is sure to become a family favorite!

25. Cauliflower Steaks with Chimichurri Sauce

Ingredients:

For the Chimichurri Sauce:
- 1 cup fresh parsley leaves, finely chopped
- 1/4 cup fresh cilantro leaves, finely chopped
- 3 cloves garlic, minced
- 2 tablespoons red wine vinegar or white wine vinegar
- 1/4 cup extra virgin olive oil
- 1/2 teaspoon dried oregano
- 1/4 teaspoon red pepper flakes (adjust to taste)
- Salt and pepper to taste

For the Cauliflower Steaks:
- 1 large head of cauliflower
- 2-3 tablespoons olive oil
- Salt and pepper to taste
- Optional: smoked paprika, garlic powder, or other seasonings of your choice

Instructions:

For the Cauliflower Steaks:
1. Preheat your oven to 425°F (220°C).
2. Remove the leaves and trim the stem of the cauliflower, leaving the core intact.
3. Place the cauliflower head upright on a cutting board and slice it into 1-inch thick slices, creating cauliflower steaks. You should get 2-3 steaks from one head of cauliflower, depending on the size.
4. Brush both sides of each cauliflower steak with olive oil and season with salt, pepper, and any additional seasonings of your choice, such as smoked paprika or garlic powder.
5. Place the cauliflower steaks on a baking sheet lined with parchment paper or aluminum foil.
6. Roast the cauliflower steaks in the preheated oven for 25-30 minutes, or until golden brown and tender, flipping halfway through cooking for even browning.

For the Chimichurri Sauce:
1. In a small bowl, combine the finely chopped parsley, cilantro, minced garlic, red wine vinegar, extra virgin olive oil, dried oregano, and red pepper flakes.
2. Season the chimichurri sauce with salt and pepper to taste. Adjust the amount of red pepper flakes based on your desired level of spiciness.
3. Stir the ingredients together until well combined. Taste and adjust the seasoning if needed.

Assembly:
1. Once the cauliflower steaks are roasted and tender, transfer them to serving plates.
2. Spoon the chimichurri sauce over the cauliflower steaks, dividing it evenly among them.
3. Serve the cauliflower steaks with chimichurri sauce immediately, alongside your favorite side dishes.

26. Sweet Potato and Spinach Quesadillas

Ingredients:
- 4 large flour tortillas
- 1 tablespoon olive oil
- Salt and pepper to taste
- Optional: salsa, sour cream, or guacamole for serving
- 2 medium sweet potatoes, peeled and diced
- 2 cups fresh spinach leaves
- 1 cup shredded cheese (cheddar, Monterey Jack, or your choice)

Instructions:

1. Boil or steam the diced sweet potatoes until they are tender, about 10-15 minutes. Drain and set aside.

2. In a large skillet, heat olive oil over medium heat. Add the cooked sweet potatoes to the skillet and cook for 2-3 minutes, stirring occasionally, until lightly browned.

3. Add the fresh spinach leaves to the skillet with the sweet potatoes. Cook for another 1-2 minutes, stirring, until the spinach is wilted. Season with salt and pepper to taste.

4. Remove the sweet potato and spinach mixture from the skillet and set aside.

5. In the same skillet (or a separate skillet if preferred), place one flour tortilla. Sprinkle a layer of shredded cheese over half of the tortilla.

6. Spoon some of the sweet potato and spinach mixture over the cheese.

7. Fold the empty half of the tortilla over the filling, creating a half-moon shape.

8. Cook the quesadilla for 2-3 minutes on each side, or until golden brown and the cheese is melted.

9. Repeat the process with the remaining tortillas and filling ingredients.

10. Once all the quesadillas are cooked, remove them from the skillet and slice each one into wedges.

11. Serve the sweet potato and spinach quesadillas hot, with salsa, sour cream, or guacamole on the side for dipping, if desired. Enjoy your delicious and nutritious quesadillas as a satisfying meal or snack!

Feel free to customize the quesadillas by adding other ingredients such as black beans, corn, onions, or bell peppers. They're versatile and perfect for using up leftover vegetables in your fridge.

27. Three Bean Salad

Ingredients:
- 1 can (15 ounces) kidney beans, drained and rinsed
- 1 can (15 ounces) cannellini beans, drained and rinsed
- 1 can (15 ounces) black beans, drained and rinsed
- 1/2 red onion, finely chopped
- 1 bell pepper (any color), diced
- 1/4 cup chopped fresh parsley or cilantro
- 1/4 cup olive oil
- 1/4 cup apple cider vinegar or red wine vinegar
- 1 tablespoon maple syrup or honey (optional)
- 1 teaspoon Dijon mustard
- Salt and pepper to taste

Instructions:
1. In a large mixing bowl, combine the drained and rinsed kidney beans, cannellini beans, and black beans.

2. Add the finely chopped red onion, diced bell pepper, and chopped fresh parsley or cilantro to the bowl with the beans.

3. In a small bowl, whisk together the olive oil, apple cider vinegar or red wine vinegar, maple syrup or honey (if using), Dijon mustard, salt, and pepper to make the dressing.

4. Pour the dressing over the bean mixture in the large bowl.

5. Toss everything together until well combined and evenly coated with the dressing.

6. Taste and adjust the seasoning, adding more salt and pepper if needed.

7. Cover the bowl and refrigerate the three bean salad for at least 1 hour before serving to allow the flavors to meld together.

8. Before serving, give the salad a quick toss to redistribute the dressing.

9. Serve the three bean salad chilled as a refreshing side dish or light meal. Enjoy the delicious combination of flavors and textures in this classic bean salad!

Feel free to customize the salad by adding other ingredients such as chopped tomatoes, corn kernels, diced avocado, or sliced olives. It's a versatile dish that's perfect for picnics, barbecues, potlucks, or as a healthy lunch option.

28. Roasted Vegetable Quinoa Bowls

Ingredients:
- 1 cup quinoa, rinsed
- 2 cups water or vegetable broth
- 2 cups mixed vegetables (such as bell peppers, zucchini, carrots, broccoli, or cauliflower), chopped into bite-sized pieces
- 2 tablespoons olive oil
- 1 teaspoon dried herbs (such as thyme, rosemary, or oregano)
- Salt and pepper to taste
- Optional toppings: avocado slices, crumbled feta or goat cheese, toasted nuts or seeds, fresh herbs, or a drizzle of balsamic glaze

Instructions:
1. Preheat your oven to 425°F (220°C).

2. In a medium saucepan, combine the rinsed quinoa and water or vegetable broth. Bring to a boil, then reduce the heat to low, cover, and simmer for 15-20 minutes, or until the quinoa is cooked and the liquid is absorbed. Remove from heat and let it sit, covered, for 5 minutes. Fluff the quinoa with a fork and set aside.

3. Meanwhile, spread the chopped mixed vegetables out on a baking sheet lined with parchment paper or aluminum foil.

4. Drizzle the vegetables with olive oil and sprinkle with dried herbs, salt, and pepper. Toss to coat evenly.

5. Roast the vegetables in the preheated oven for 20-25 minutes, or until they are tender and lightly browned, stirring halfway through cooking for even browning.

6. Once the vegetables are roasted, divide the cooked quinoa among serving bowls.

7. Top each bowl of quinoa with a portion of the roasted vegetables.

8. If desired, add optional toppings such as avocado slices, crumbled feta or goat cheese, toasted nuts or seeds, fresh herbs, or a drizzle of balsamic glaze.

9. Serve the roasted vegetable quinoa bowls hot, and enjoy the delicious and nutritious combination of flavors and textures!

Feel free to customize these quinoa bowls with your favorite vegetables and toppings. They're a versatile and satisfying meal option that's perfect for lunch or dinner.

29. Lentil Veggie Burgers

Ingredients:
- 1 cup cooked lentils (green or brown)
- 1 cup cooked quinoa
- 1/2 cup finely chopped onion
- 1/2 cup grated carrot
- 1/2 cup finely chopped bell pepper (any color)
- 2 cloves garlic, minced
- 1/4 cup breadcrumbs
- 2 tablespoons ground flaxseed meal
- 3 tablespoons water
- 1 teaspoon smoked paprika
- 1 teaspoon ground cumin
- Salt and pepper to taste
- Olive oil for cooking

Instructions:

1. Preheat your oven to 375°F (190°C).

2. In a small bowl, mix together ground flaxseed meal and water. Let it sit for a few minutes to thicken and form a gel-like consistency.

3. In a large mixing bowl, combine the cooked lentils, cooked quinoa, finely chopped onion, grated carrot, chopped bell pepper, minced garlic, breadcrumbs, smoked paprika, ground cumin, salt, and pepper.

4. Add the flaxseed mixture to the bowl and mix everything together until well combined.

5. Using your hands, shape the mixture into patties of your desired size and thickness.

6. Heat a small amount of olive oil in a skillet over medium heat. Once hot, add the lentil veggie patties to the skillet (you may need to cook them in batches depending on the size of your skillet).

7. Cook the patties for 3-4 minutes on each side, or until they are golden brown and heated through.

8. Transfer the cooked lentil veggie burgers to a baking sheet lined with parchment paper or aluminum foil.

9. Bake the burgers in the preheated oven for an additional 10-15 minutes to ensure they are cooked through and firm.

10. Once done, remove the lentil veggie burgers from the oven and let them cool slightly before serving.

11. Serve the lentil veggie burgers on buns with your favorite toppings such as lettuce, tomato, onion, avocado, and condiments.

12. Enjoy your homemade lentil veggie burgers as a delicious and nutritious plant-based meal option

30. Grilled Portobello Mushroom Fajitas

Ingredients:
- 4 large portobello mushrooms, stems removed and sliced
- 2 bell peppers, thinly sliced
- 1 onion, thinly sliced
- 3 tablespoons olive oil
- 2 cloves garlic, minced
- 2 teaspoons chili powder
- 1 teaspoon ground cumin
- 1 teaspoon smoked paprika
- Salt and pepper to taste
- 8 small flour tortillas
- Optional toppings: sliced avocado, salsa, sour cream, shredded cheese, chopped cilantro, lime wedges

Instructions:

1. Preheat your grill to medium-high heat.

2. In a large bowl, toss the sliced portobello mushrooms, bell peppers, and onion with olive oil, minced garlic, chili powder, ground cumin, smoked paprika, salt, and pepper until well coated.

3. Place the seasoned vegetables on the preheated grill and cook for 5-6 minutes per side, or until they are tender and lightly charred. Remove from the grill and set aside.

4. While the vegetables are grilling, warm the flour tortillas on the grill for about 30 seconds per side, or until they are heated through and lightly charred.

5. Once the vegetables and tortillas are cooked, assemble the fajitas by placing a spoonful of the grilled vegetable mixture onto each tortilla.

6. Add your desired toppings such as sliced avocado, salsa, sour cream, shredded cheese, chopped cilantro, and a squeeze of lime juice.

7. Fold the tortillas over the filling and serve the grilled portobello mushroom fajitas immediately.

8. Enjoy the delicious flavors and textures of these vegetarian fajitas as a satisfying and wholesome meal!

Feel free to customize the fajitas with additional toppings or seasonings to suit your taste preferences. They're perfect for a quick and easy weeknight dinner or for entertaining guests at a summer barbecue.

31. Roasted Garlic Hummus with Veggies

Ingredients:

For the Roasted Garlic Hummus:
- 1 can (15 ounces) chickpeas, drained and rinsed
- 3 tablespoons tahini
- 3 tablespoons lemon juice (about 1 lemon)
- 2 tablespoons extra virgin olive oil
- 2 cloves roasted garlic (or 1-2 cloves raw garlic, minced)
- 1/2 teaspoon ground cumin
- Salt to taste
- Water (as needed to adjust consistency)

For the Veggie Platter:
- Assorted fresh vegetables (such as carrot sticks, cucumber slices, bell pepper strips, cherry tomatoes, celery sticks, and snap peas)

Instructions:

For the Roasted Garlic Hummus:

1. If you're using raw garlic, mince it finely and set it aside. If you're using roasted garlic, squeeze the roasted cloves out of their skins and set them aside.

2. In a food processor, combine the chickpeas, tahini, lemon juice, olive oil, roasted or raw garlic, ground cumin, and a pinch of salt.

3. Blend the ingredients until smooth, stopping to scrape down the sides of the bowl as needed. If the hummus is too thick, you can add water, a tablespoon at a time, until you reach your desired consistency.

4. Taste the hummus and adjust the seasoning, adding more salt or lemon juice if needed.

For the Veggie Platter:

1. Wash and prepare your assorted fresh vegetables by cutting them into bite-sized pieces or strips.

2. Arrange the vegetable sticks and slices on a platter around a bowl of the roasted garlic hummus.

3. Serve the roasted garlic hummus with veggies as a healthy and flavorful snack or appetizer.

Feel free to customize your roasted garlic hummus with additional ingredients such as roasted red pepper, sun-dried tomatoes, or fresh herbs like parsley or cilantro. Enjoy dipping your favorite veggies into this creamy and flavorful hummus for a satisfying and nutritious snack!

32. Vegetable Stir-Fry with Tofu

Ingredients:
- 14 oz (400g) firm tofu, pressed and cubed
- 2 tablespoons soy sauce
- 1 tablespoon sesame oil
- 2 tablespoons cornstarch
- 2 tablespoons vegetable oil
- 2 cloves garlic, minced
- 1 tablespoon minced ginger
- 1 onion, sliced mushrooms, etc.), sliced
- Salt and pepper to taste
- Cooked rice or noodles for serving
- 2 cups mixed vegetables (such as bell peppers, broccoli, carrots, snap peas,

Sauce:
- 1/4 cup soy sauce
- 2 tablespoons hoisin sauce
- 1 tablespoon rice vinegar
- 1 tablespoon brown sugar
- 1 teaspoon sriracha or chili sauce (adjust to taste)
- 1 teaspoon cornstarch mixed with 1 tablespoon water

Instructions:
1. In a bowl, combine the cubed tofu with soy sauce, sesame oil, and cornstarch. Toss gently to coat the tofu evenly.

2. Heat vegetable oil in a large skillet or wok over medium-high heat. Add the tofu cubes and cook until golden brown on all sides. Remove from the skillet and set aside.

3. In the same skillet, add a bit more oil if needed. Add minced garlic and ginger, and sauté for about 1 minute until fragrant.

4. Add sliced onion and cook for 2-3 minutes until softened.

5. Add the mixed vegetables to the skillet and stir-fry for 3-4 minutes until they are tender-crisp.

6. In a small bowl, whisk together the sauce ingredients: soy sauce, hoisin sauce, rice vinegar, brown sugar, sriracha, and cornstarch mixture. Pour the sauce over the vegetables in the skillet.

7. Return the cooked tofu to the skillet and toss everything together until the sauce thickens and coats the tofu and vegetables.

8. Season with salt and pepper to taste. Serve the vegetable stir-fry with tofu over cooked rice or noodles. Garnish with sliced green onions and sesame seeds if desired. Enjoy your delicious and nutritious vegetable stir-fry with tofu!

Feel free to customize this stir-fry with your favorite vegetables and adjust the sauce to your taste preferences. It's a versatile and satisfying dish that's perfect for a quick and healthy meal.

33. Kale and White Bean Soup

Ingredients:
- 1 tablespoon olive oil
- 1 onion, chopped
- 2 carrots, diced
- 2 celery stalks, diced
- 3 cloves garlic, minced
- 4 cups vegetable broth
- Salt and pepper to taste
- Optional toppings: grated Parmesan cheese, red pepper flakes, crusty bread
- 2 cans (15 ounces each) white beans (such as cannellini or Great Northern), drained and rinsed
- 1 bunch kale, stems removed and leaves chopped
- 1 teaspoon dried thyme
- 1 teaspoon dried rosemary

Instructions:

1. In a large pot, heat the olive oil over medium heat. Add the chopped onion, diced carrots, and diced celery. Cook, stirring occasionally, until the vegetables are softened, about 5-7 minutes.

2. Add the minced garlic to the pot and cook for an additional 1-2 minutes, until fragrant.

3. Pour in the vegetable broth and bring the soup to a simmer.

4. Stir in the drained and rinsed white beans, chopped kale leaves, dried thyme, and dried rosemary.

5. Reduce the heat to low, cover the pot, and let the soup simmer for about 15-20 minutes, or until the kale is tender and wilted.

6. Once the kale is cooked, season the soup with salt and pepper to taste, adjusting as needed.

7. If you prefer a thicker soup, you can use an immersion blender to partially blend the soup, leaving some beans and vegetables whole for texture.

8. Serve the kale and white bean soup hot, garnished with grated Parmesan cheese, red pepper flakes, and accompanied by crusty bread for dipping. Enjoy the warm and comforting flavors of this hearty soup!

Feel free to customize this soup by adding other vegetables such as diced potatoes or tomatoes, or by incorporating your favorite herbs and spices. It's a versatile and satisfying dish that's perfect for a cozy meal any time of year.

34. Roasted Sweet Potato and Arugula Salad

Ingredients:
- 2 medium sweet potatoes, peeled and diced into cubes
- 2 tablespoons olive oil
- 1 teaspoon smoked paprika
- 1/2 teaspoon ground cumin
- Salt and pepper to taste
- 4 cups arugula leaves, washed and dried
- 1/4 cup dried cranberries or raisins
- 1/4 cup toasted pecans or walnuts, chopped
- 1/4 cup crumbled feta cheese or goat cheese (optional)

For the Dressing:
- 2 tablespoons balsamic vinegar
- 1 tablespoon maple syrup or honey
- 2 tablespoons extra virgin olive oil
- Salt and pepper to taste

Instructions:

1. Preheat your oven to 400°F (200°C).

2. In a large mixing bowl, toss the diced sweet potatoes with olive oil, smoked paprika, ground cumin, salt, and pepper until evenly coated.

3. Spread the seasoned sweet potatoes out in a single layer on a baking sheet lined with parchment paper or aluminum foil.

4. Roast the sweet potatoes in the preheated oven for 20-25 minutes, or until they are tender and lightly caramelized, stirring halfway through cooking for even browning.

5. While the sweet potatoes are roasting, prepare the dressing by whisking together balsamic vinegar, maple syrup or honey, extra virgin olive oil, salt, and pepper in a small bowl. Set aside.

6. Once the sweet potatoes are roasted, remove them from the oven and let them cool slightly.

7. In a large serving bowl, combine the arugula leaves, roasted sweet potatoes, dried cranberries or raisins, and toasted pecans or walnuts.

8. Drizzle the dressing over the salad and toss everything together until evenly coated.

9. If using, sprinkle crumbled feta cheese or goat cheese over the top of the salad.

10. Serve the roasted sweet potato and arugula salad immediately as a delicious and nutritious side dish or light meal. Enjoy the vibrant flavors and textures of this delightful salad!

35. Veggie-Packed Omelets

Ingredients:
- 3 large eggs
- 1/4 cup milk or water
- Salt and pepper to taste
- 1 tablespoon butter or olive oil
- 1/4 cup diced onion
- 1/4 cup diced bell pepper (any color)
- 1/4 cup diced tomato
- 1/4 cup sliced mushrooms
- 1/4 cup chopped spinach or kale
- 1/4 cup shredded cheese (such as cheddar, mozzarella, or feta)
- Optional toppings: avocado slices, salsa, sour cream, chopped fresh herbs

Instructions:

1. In a bowl, whisk together the eggs, milk or water, salt, and pepper until well combined.

2. Heat the butter or olive oil in a non-stick skillet over medium heat.

3. Add the diced onion, bell pepper, tomato, mushrooms, and chopped spinach or kale to the skillet. Cook for 2-3 minutes, or until the vegetables are softened.

4. Pour the whisked egg mixture over the cooked vegetables in the skillet.

5. Using a spatula, gently lift the edges of the omelet as it cooks, allowing the uncooked eggs to flow underneath.

6. When the omelet is mostly set but still slightly runny on top, sprinkle the shredded cheese evenly over one half of the omelet.

7. Fold the other half of the omelet over the cheese to enclose the filling, creating a half-moon shape.

8. Cook the omelet for another 1-2 minutes, or until the cheese is melted and the eggs are fully cooked through.

9. Slide the omelet onto a plate and garnish with optional toppings such as avocado slices, salsa, sour cream, or chopped fresh herbs. Serve the veggie-packed omelet hot, and enjoy a nutritious and satisfying breakfast!

Feel free to customize your omelet with your favorite vegetables, cheese, and toppings. It's a versatile dish that's perfect for using up leftover vegetables in your fridge and for starting your day on a healthy note.

36. Black Bean and Quinoa Burrito Bowls

Ingredients:
- 1 cup quinoa, rinsed
- 2 cups water or vegetable broth
- 1 tablespoon olive oil
- 1 onion, diced
- 2 cloves garlic, minced
- 1 bell pepper, diced
- 1 can (15 ounces) black beans, drained and rinsed
- 1 cup corn kernels (fresh, frozen, or canned)
- 1 teaspoon ground cumin
- 1 teaspoon chili powder
- Salt and pepper to taste
- Juice of 1 lime
- Optional toppings: diced avocado or guacamole, salsa, shredded cheese, chopped cilantro, sour cream or Greek yogurt, lime wedges

Instructions:

1. In a medium saucepan, combine the rinsed quinoa and water or vegetable broth. Bring to a boil, then reduce the heat to low, cover, and simmer for 15-20 minutes, or until the quinoa is cooked and the liquid is absorbed. Remove from heat and let it sit, covered, for 5 minutes. Fluff the quinoa with a fork and set aside.

2. While the quinoa is cooking, heat olive oil in a large skillet over medium heat. Add diced onion and cook for 3-4 minutes until softened.

3. Add minced garlic and diced bell pepper to the skillet and cook for an additional 2-3 minutes until fragrant and the vegetables are tender.

4. Stir in the drained and rinsed black beans, corn kernels, ground cumin, and chili powder. Cook for 2-3 minutes until heated through.

5. Season the black bean and vegetable mixture with salt, pepper, and lime juice. Adjust seasoning to taste.

6. To assemble the burrito bowls, divide the cooked quinoa among serving bowls.

7. Top the quinoa with the black bean and vegetable mixture.

8. Add your desired toppings such as diced avocado or guacamole, salsa, shredded cheese, chopped cilantro, sour cream or Greek yogurt, and lime wedges.

9. Serve the black bean and quinoa burrito bowls immediately and enjoy!

Feel free to customize your burrito bowls with additional toppings such as sliced jalapeños, diced tomatoes, shredded lettuce, or hot sauce. It's a versatile and satisfying meal that's perfect for lunch or dinner.

37. Mediterranean Grilled Vegetables

Ingredients:
- 1 medium eggplant, sliced into rounds
- 2 medium zucchini, sliced into rounds
- 1 red bell pepper, sliced into strips
- 1 yellow bell pepper, sliced into strips
- 1 red onion, sliced into rounds
- 2 tablespoons olive oil
- 2 cloves garlic, minced
- 1 teaspoon dried oregano
- 1 teaspoon dried thyme
- Salt and pepper to taste
- Juice of 1 lemon
- Fresh parsley or basil leaves for garnish (optional)

Instructions:
1. Preheat your grill to medium-high heat.

2. In a large mixing bowl, toss the sliced eggplant, zucchini, bell peppers, and red onion with olive oil, minced garlic, dried oregano, dried thyme, salt, and pepper until evenly coated.

3. Place the seasoned vegetables on the preheated grill grates in a single layer. You may need to cook them in batches depending on the size of your grill.

4. Grill the vegetables for 5-7 minutes per side, or until they are tender and lightly charred, turning them halfway through cooking for even grilling.

5. Once the vegetables are grilled to your desired level of doneness, remove them from the grill and transfer them to a serving platter.

6. Drizzle the grilled vegetables with fresh lemon juice and garnish with fresh parsley or basil leaves if desired.

7. Serve the Mediterranean grilled vegetables hot or at room temperature as a delicious side dish or appetizer.

These Mediterranean grilled vegetables are bursting with flavor and can be served alongside grilled meats, fish, or tofu, or enjoyed on their own as a vegetarian main course. They're a versatile and healthy addition to any meal!

38. Baked Falafel Bites

Ingredients:
- 1 can (15 ounces) chickpeas, drained and rinsed
- 1/4 cup fresh parsley, chopped
- 1/4 cup fresh cilantro, chopped
- 1/2 small onion, chopped
- 2 cloves garlic, minced
- 1 teaspoon ground cumin
- 1 teaspoon ground coriander
- 1/2 teaspoon baking powder
- Salt and pepper to taste
- 2 tablespoons olive oil
- Tahini sauce or yogurt sauce for serving (optional)

Instructions:
1. Preheat your oven to 375°F (190°C). Line a baking sheet with parchment paper or lightly grease it with olive oil.

2. In a food processor, combine the drained and rinsed chickpeas, chopped parsley, chopped cilantro, chopped onion, minced garlic, ground cumin, ground coriander, baking powder, salt, and pepper.

3. Pulse the ingredients together until they form a coarse paste. You may need to stop and scrape down the sides of the food processor bowl a few times to ensure everything is evenly mixed.

4. Using your hands, roll the falafel mixture into small balls, about 1 inch in diameter, and place them on the prepared baking sheet.

5. Once all the falafel balls are formed, lightly brush them with olive oil to help them brown in the oven.

6. Bake the falafel bites in the preheated oven for 20-25 minutes, or until they are golden brown and crispy on the outside, flipping them halfway through cooking for even browning.

7. Once the falafel bites are baked, remove them from the oven and let them cool slightly before serving.

8. Serve the baked falafel bites warm with tahini sauce or yogurt sauce for dipping, if desired.

These baked falafel bites are a healthier alternative to traditional fried falafel and are packed with flavor from the fresh herbs and spices. Enjoy them as a tasty snack, appetizer, or as part of a Mediterranean-inspired meal!

39. Roasted Cauliflower and Chickpea Curry

Ingredients:
- 1 head cauliflower, cut into florets
- 1 can (15 ounces) chickpeas, drained and rinsed
- 2 tablespoons olive oil
- 1 onion, chopped
- 3 cloves garlic, minced
- 1 tablespoon grated ginger
- 2 tablespoons curry powder
- 1 teaspoon ground cumin
- 1 teaspoon ground coriander
- 1/2 teaspoon turmeric powder
- 1 can (14 ounces) diced tomatoes
- 1 can (14 ounces) coconut milk
- Salt and pepper to taste
- Fresh cilantro leaves for garnish (optional)
- Cooked rice or naan bread for serving

Instructions:

1. Preheat your oven to 400°F (200°C).

2. In a large bowl, toss the cauliflower florets and chickpeas with 1 tablespoon of olive oil until evenly coated. Spread them out on a baking sheet lined with parchment paper or aluminum foil.

3. Roast the cauliflower and chickpeas in the preheated oven for 20-25 minutes, or until they are tender and golden brown, stirring halfway through cooking for even browning.

4. While the cauliflower and chickpeas are roasting, heat the remaining 1 tablespoon of olive oil in a large skillet or pot over medium heat.

5. Add the chopped onion to the skillet and cook for 3-4 minutes until softened.

6. Stir in the minced garlic and grated ginger, and cook for an additional 1-2 minutes until fragrant.

7. Add the curry powder, ground cumin, ground coriander, and turmeric powder to the skillet, and cook for 1 minute, stirring constantly, until the spices are fragrant.

8. Pour in the diced tomatoes (with their juices) and coconut milk, and stir to combine. Bring the mixture to a simmer.

9. Once the cauliflower and chickpeas are roasted, add them to the skillet with the curry sauce, and stir to coat them in the sauce. Season with salt and pepper to taste.

10. Let the curry simmer for 5-10 minutes to allow the flavors to meld together and the sauce to thicken slightly.

11. Serve the roasted cauliflower and chickpea curry hot, garnished with fresh cilantro leaves if desired. Serve with cooked rice or naan bread on the side

40. Vegetable Stuffed Portobello Mushrooms

Ingredients:
- 4 large portobello mushrooms, stems removed
- 2 tablespoons olive oil
- 2 cloves garlic, minced
- 1 small onion, finely chopped
- 1 bell pepper, diced
- 1 zucchini, diced
- 1 cup cherry tomatoes, halved
- 1 cup baby spinach, chopped
- 1/4 cup grated Parmesan cheese (optional)
- Salt and pepper to taste
- Fresh herbs (such as basil or parsley) for garnish

Instructions:

1. Preheat your oven to 375°F (190°C). Line a baking sheet with parchment paper.

2. Clean the portobello mushrooms by wiping them with a damp cloth or paper towel. Remove the stems and gently scrape out the gills using a spoon.

3. In a large skillet, heat the olive oil over medium heat. Add the minced garlic and chopped onion, and sauté for 2-3 minutes until softened and fragrant.

4. Add the diced bell pepper and zucchini to the skillet, and cook for another 5 minutes until the vegetables are tender.

5. Stir in the cherry tomatoes and chopped spinach, and cook for an additional 2-3 minutes until the spinach is wilted and the tomatoes are softened.

6. Season the vegetable mixture with salt and pepper to taste. Remove the skillet from the heat.

7. Place the portobello mushrooms on the prepared baking sheet, gill-side up.

8. Divide the vegetable mixture evenly among the portobello mushrooms, spooning it into the mushroom caps.

9. If using, sprinkle grated Parmesan cheese over the stuffed mushrooms for added flavor.

10. Bake the stuffed portobello mushrooms in the preheated oven for 15-20 minutes, or until the mushrooms are tender and the filling is heated through.

11. Once done, remove the mushrooms from the oven and garnish with fresh herbs before serving.

12. Serve the vegetable-stuffed portobello mushrooms hot as a delicious and nutritious main course or appetizer.

41. Avocado and Black Bean Salad

Ingredients:
- 2 ripe avocados, diced
- 1 can (15 ounces) black beans, drained and rinsed
- 1 cup cherry tomatoes, halved
- 1/4 cup red onion, finely chopped
- 1/4 cup fresh cilantro, chopped
- 1 jalapeño pepper, seeded and diced (optional, for heat)
- Juice of 1 lime
- 2 tablespoons olive oil
- Salt and pepper to taste

Instructions:

1. In a large mixing bowl, combine the diced avocados, black beans, halved cherry tomatoes, chopped red onion, chopped cilantro, and diced jalapeño pepper (if using).

2. In a small bowl, whisk together the lime juice, olive oil, salt, and pepper to make the dressing.

3. Pour the dressing over the avocado and black bean mixture in the large bowl.

4. Gently toss everything together until well combined and evenly coated with the dressing.

5. Taste and adjust the seasoning, adding more salt and pepper if needed.

6. Cover the bowl and refrigerate the avocado and black bean salad for at least 30 minutes to allow the flavors to meld together.

7. Before serving, give the salad a quick toss to redistribute the dressing.

8. Serve the avocado and black bean salad chilled as a refreshing side dish or light meal.

This avocado and black bean salad is packed with creamy avocado, protein-rich black beans, and fresh vegetables, all tossed in a zesty lime dressing. It's a vibrant and flavorful dish that's perfect for picnics, barbecues, potlucks, or as a healthy lunch option. Enjoy the delicious combination of flavors and textures in this simple and satisfying salad!

42. Grilled Vegetable Skewers

Ingredients:
- Assorted vegetables, such as bell peppers, zucchini, cherry tomatoes, red onion, mushrooms, and yellow squash
- Olive oil
- Balsamic vinegar (optional)
- Garlic powder
- Italian seasoning or dried herbs of your choice
- Salt and pepper to taste
- Wooden or metal skewers

Instructions:

1. If you're using wooden skewers, soak them in water for at least 30 minutes to prevent them from burning on the grill.

2. Prepare the vegetables by washing them and cutting them into bite-sized pieces.

3. In a large bowl, toss the vegetables with olive oil, a splash of balsamic vinegar (if desired), garlic powder, Italian seasoning or dried herbs, salt, and pepper. Make sure the vegetables are evenly coated with the seasoning mixture.

4. Thread the seasoned vegetables onto the skewers, alternating between different types of vegetables to create colorful skewers.

5. Preheat your grill to medium-high heat.

6. Place the vegetable skewers on the preheated grill and cook for 8-10 minutes, turning occasionally, until the vegetables are tender and slightly charred.

7. Once the vegetable skewers are cooked to your liking, remove them from the grill and serve immediately.

8. Optional: Garnish the grilled vegetable skewers with fresh herbs, a drizzle of balsamic glaze, or a sprinkle of grated Parmesan cheese before serving.

These grilled vegetable skewers are versatile and can be customized with your favorite vegetables and seasonings. They're a healthy and flavorful side dish or vegetarian option for summer gatherings or weeknight dinners. Enjoy the delicious flavors of grilled vegetables straight from the barbecue!

43. Lentil and Sweet Potato Stew

Ingredients:
- 1 tablespoon olive oil
- 1 onion, chopped
- 2 cloves garlic, minced
- 2 medium sweet potatoes, peeled and diced
- 1 cup dry brown lentils, rinsed and drained
- 4 cups vegetable broth or water
- 1 can (14 ounces) diced tomatoes
- 1 teaspoon ground cumin
- 1 teaspoon ground coriander
- 1/2 teaspoon smoked paprika
- Salt and pepper to taste
- 2 cups chopped kale or spinach
- Juice of 1 lemon
- Fresh parsley or cilantro for garnish (optional)

Instructions:

1. Heat the olive oil in a large pot or Dutch oven over medium heat. Add the chopped onion and cook for 3-4 minutes until softened.

2. Add the minced garlic to the pot and cook for an additional 1-2 minutes until fragrant.

3. Stir in the diced sweet potatoes, dry brown lentils, vegetable broth or water, diced tomatoes (with their juices), ground cumin, ground coriander, smoked paprika, salt, and pepper.

4. Bring the stew to a boil, then reduce the heat to low and let it simmer, partially covered, for 20-25 minutes, or until the sweet potatoes and lentils are tender.

5. Once the sweet potatoes and lentils are cooked through, stir in the chopped kale or spinach and let it simmer for an additional 5 minutes until wilted.

6. Remove the pot from the heat and stir in the lemon juice. Taste and adjust the seasoning, adding more salt and pepper if needed.

7. Ladle the lentil and sweet potato stew into bowls and garnish with fresh parsley or cilantro if desired. Serve the stew hot, and enjoy the hearty and comforting flavors!

This lentil and sweet potato stew is nutritious, filling, and packed with flavor. It's a satisfying meal on its own, or you can serve it with crusty bread or rice for a complete and comforting dinner.

44. Roasted Beet and Orange Salad

Ingredients:
- 3 medium beets, peeled and diced
- 2 oranges, peeled and segmented
- 2 tablespoons balsamic vinegar
- 2 tablespoons extra virgin olive oil
- Salt and pepper to taste
- 4 cups mixed salad greens (such as spinach, arugula, or mixed baby greens)
- 1/4 cup crumbled feta cheese or goat cheese (optional)
- 1/4 cup chopped walnuts or pecans, toasted (optional)

Instructions:
1. Preheat your oven to 400°F (200°C). Line a baking sheet with parchment paper or aluminum foil.

2. Place the diced beets on the prepared baking sheet and drizzle with a little olive oil. Season with salt and pepper to taste, and toss to coat the beets evenly.

3. Roast the beets in the preheated oven for 25-30 minutes, or until tender when pierced with a fork. Remove from the oven and let them cool slightly.

4. While the beets are roasting, prepare the oranges by peeling them and segmenting them. Set aside.

5. In a small bowl, whisk together the balsamic vinegar and extra virgin olive oil to make the dressing. Season with salt and pepper to taste.

6. Arrange the mixed salad greens on a serving platter or individual plates.

7. Top the greens with the roasted beets and orange segments.

8. If using, sprinkle crumbled feta cheese or goat cheese and chopped toasted walnuts or pecans over the salad.

9. Drizzle the balsamic vinaigrette over the salad just before serving.

10. Optional: Garnish with additional fresh herbs or citrus zest for extra flavor and color.

11. Serve the roasted beet and orange salad immediately as a refreshing and colorful appetizer or side dish.

This roasted beet and orange salad is not only visually stunning but also bursting with flavor and nutrients. Enjoy the combination of sweet roasted beets, juicy oranges, and tangy dressing in every bite!

45. Tofu Vegetable Lettuce Wraps

Ingredients:
- 1 block (14 ounces) firm tofu, drained and pressed
- 2 tablespoons soy sauce or tamari
- 1 tablespoon rice vinegar
- 1 tablespoon sesame oil
- 1 tablespoon hoisin sauce
- 2 teaspoons cornstarch
- 1 tablespoon vegetable oil
- 2 cloves garlic, minced
- 1 teaspoon grated ginger
- 1 small onion, finely chopped
- 1 bell pepper, diced
- 1 carrot, grated
- 1 cup chopped mushrooms (such as shiitake or cremini)
- 1/4 cup chopped water chestnuts
- 1/4 cup chopped green onions
- Salt and pepper to taste
- 1 head butter lettuce or iceberg lettuce, leaves separated

Instructions:

1. Start by preparing the tofu. Cut the pressed tofu into small cubes and set aside.

2. In a small bowl, whisk together the soy sauce or tamari, rice vinegar, sesame oil, hoisin sauce, and cornstarch to make the sauce. Set aside.

3. Heat vegetable oil in a large skillet or wok over medium-high heat. Add the minced garlic and grated ginger, and sauté for 1-2 minutes until fragrant.

4. Add the chopped onion, diced bell pepper, grated carrot, and chopped mushrooms to the skillet. Cook for 5-6 minutes until the vegetables are softened.

5. Add the chopped tofu to the skillet and cook for an additional 3-4 minutes, stirring occasionally, until the tofu is lightly browned.

6. Pour the sauce over the tofu and vegetable mixture in the skillet. Stir well to coat everything evenly with the sauce.

7. Cook for another 2-3 minutes until the sauce has thickened slightly.

8. Stir in the chopped water chestnuts and chopped green onions. Season with salt and pepper to taste.

9. To assemble the lettuce wraps, spoon the tofu and vegetable mixture onto individual lettuce leaves.

10. Serve the tofu vegetable lettuce wraps immediately, and enjoy the delicious combination of flavors and textures!

46. Cauliflower Fried Rice

Ingredients:
- 1 medium head cauliflower
- 2 tablespoons vegetable oil or sesame oil
- 2 cloves garlic, minced
- 1 small onion, finely chopped
- 1 carrot, diced
- 1 cup frozen peas and carrots mix
- 2 eggs, lightly beaten
- 3 tablespoons soy sauce or tamari
- 1 tablespoon oyster sauce (optional)
- 1 teaspoon toasted sesame oil (optional)
- Salt and pepper to taste
- Chopped green onions for garnish
- Sesame seeds for garnish (optional)

Instructions:

1. Cut the cauliflower into florets and pulse them in a food processor until they resemble rice grains. You can also use a box grater to grate the cauliflower.

2. Heat 1 tablespoon of vegetable oil or sesame oil in a large skillet or wok over medium heat.

3. Add the minced garlic and chopped onion to the skillet, and sauté for 2-3 minutes until fragrant and softened.

4. Add the diced carrot and frozen peas and carrots mix to the skillet, and cook for another 3-4 minutes until the vegetables are tender.

5. Push the vegetables to one side of the skillet, and pour the beaten eggs into the empty space. Allow them to cook for a minute or two, then scramble them with a spatula until cooked through. Break them into small pieces.

6. Push the vegetables and eggs to the side of the skillet again, and add the remaining tablespoon of vegetable oil or sesame oil to the empty space.

7. Add the riced cauliflower to the skillet, and stir to combine everything together.

8. Drizzle the soy sauce or tamari, and oyster sauce (if using) over the cauliflower mixture. Stir well to evenly distribute the sauces.

9. Cook the cauliflower fried rice for 5-7 minutes, stirring occasionally, until the cauliflower is tender but not mushy.

10. Taste and adjust the seasoning with salt and pepper as needed. If desired, drizzle with toasted sesame oil for extra flavor.

11. Garnish the cauliflower fried rice with chopped green onions and sesame seeds before serving.

12. Serve the cauliflower fried rice hot as a delicious and healthy alternative to traditional fried rice!

47. Roasted Brussels Sprouts and Chickpea Salad

Ingredients:
- 1 lb Brussels sprouts, trimmed and halved
- 1 can (15 ounces) chickpeas, drained and rinsed
- 2 tablespoons olive oil
- 1 teaspoon smoked paprika
- 1/2 teaspoon garlic powder
- 1/4 cup toasted walnuts or pecans, chopped
- 2 tablespoons balsamic vinegar
- 1 tablespoon honey or maple syrup
- 2 tablespoons extra virgin olive oil
- 1 teaspoon Dijon mustard
- Salt and pepper to taste
- Salt and pepper to taste
- 1/4 cup dried cranberries or raisins
- Fresh parsley or cilantro for garnish (optional)

Instructions:

1. Preheat your oven to 400°F (200°C). Line a baking sheet with parchment paper or aluminum foil.

2. In a large mixing bowl, toss the halved Brussels sprouts and chickpeas with olive oil, smoked paprika, garlic powder, salt, and pepper until evenly coated.

3. Spread the Brussels sprouts and chickpeas out in a single layer on the prepared baking sheet.

4. Roast the Brussels sprouts and chickpeas in the preheated oven for 25-30 minutes, or until the Brussels sprouts are tender and caramelized, and the chickpeas are crispy, stirring halfway through cooking for even browning.

5. While the Brussels sprouts and chickpeas are roasting, prepare the dressing. In a small bowl, whisk together the balsamic vinegar, honey or maple syrup, extra virgin olive oil, Dijon mustard, salt, and pepper until well combined.

6. Once the Brussels sprouts and chickpeas are roasted, transfer them to a large mixing bowl. Add the dried cranberries or raisins and toasted walnuts or pecans to the bowl.

7. Drizzle the dressing over the salad and toss everything together until evenly coated. Taste and adjust the seasoning, adding more salt and pepper if needed.

8. Garnish the roasted Brussels sprouts and chickpea salad with fresh parsley or cilantro before serving, if desired. Serve the salad warm or at room temperature as a delicious and nutritious side dish or light meal.

This roasted Brussels sprouts and chickpea salad is packed with flavor and texture, making it a satisfying dish that's perfect for any occasion. Enjoy the delicious combination of sweet, savory, and crunchy flavors!

48. Quinoa and Black Bean Stuffed Peppers

Ingredients:
- 4 large bell peppers
- 1 cup quinoa
- 2 cups vegetable broth
- 1 can (15 oz) black beans
- 1 cup corn kernels
- 1 cup diced tomatoes
- 1 small onion, finely chopped
- 2 cloves garlic, minced
- 1 tsp each ground cumin and chili powder
- Salt and pepper to taste
- 1 cup shredded cheese
- Fresh cilantro or parsley for garnish (optional)

Instructions:

1. Preheat oven to 375°F (190°C).

2. Cook quinoa in vegetable broth until tender.

3. Sauté onion and garlic, then add cooked quinoa, black beans, corn, tomatoes, spices, salt, and pepper.

4. Stuff bell peppers with the mixture and top with shredded cheese.

5. Bake covered for 25-30 mins, then uncovered for 5 mins.

6. Garnish with cilantro or parsley if desired.

7. Serve hot. Enjoy your stuffed peppers!

49. Grilled Eggplant with Tomato Basil Salad

Ingredients:
- 1 large eggplant, sliced
- 2 tomatoes, diced
- 1/4 cup fresh basil leaves, chopped
- 2 tablespoons balsamic vinegar
- 2 tablespoons olive oil
- Salt and pepper to taste

Instructions:
1. Preheat grill to medium heat.

2. Brush eggplant slices with olive oil and season with salt and pepper.

3. Grill eggplant slices for 4-5 minutes per side, or until tender and grill marks appear.

4. In a bowl, combine diced tomatoes, chopped basil, balsamic vinegar, and olive oil. Season with salt and pepper to taste.

5. Serve grilled eggplant slices topped with tomato basil salad.

6. Enjoy your delicious grilled eggplant with tomato basil salad!

50. Sweet Potato and Kale Frittata

Ingredients:
- 1 large sweet potato, peeled and diced
- 2 cups kale, chopped
- 6 eggs
- 1/4 cup milk
- Salt and pepper to taste
- 1 tablespoon olive oil
- Optional: shredded cheese for topping

Instructions:
1. Preheat oven to 375°F (190°C).

2. In a skillet, heat olive oil over medium heat. Add diced sweet potato and cook until tender, about 8-10 minutes.

3. Add chopped kale to the skillet and cook until wilted, about 2-3 minutes.

4. In a bowl, whisk together eggs, milk, salt, and pepper.

5. Pour egg mixture over sweet potato and kale in the skillet.

6. Cook for 2-3 minutes until the edges start to set.

7. Transfer the skillet to the preheated oven and bake for 15-20 minutes, or until the frittata is set in the center.

8. Optional: Sprinkle shredded cheese on top and broil for an additional 2-3 minutes until cheese is melted and bubbly.

9. Remove from oven and let cool slightly before slicing.

10. Serve your delicious sweet potato and kale frittata warm.

11. Enjoy your flavorful and nutritious frittata!

51. Mediterranean Lentil Salad

Ingredients:
- 1 cup dry lentils
- 2 cups water
- 1 cucumber, diced
- 1 bell pepper, diced
- 1/2 red onion, finely chopped
- 1 cup cherry tomatoes, halved
- 1/4 cup Kalamata olives, sliced
- 1/4 cup crumbled feta cheese
- 1/4 cup chopped fresh parsley
- 2 tablespoons extra virgin olive oil
- 2 tablespoons red wine vinegar
- 1 teaspoon dried oregano
- Salt and pepper to taste

Instructions:

1. Rinse the lentils under cold water. In a saucepan, bring 2 cups of water to a boil. Add the lentils, reduce heat to low, cover, and simmer for 15-20 minutes, or until the lentils are tender but still hold their shape. Drain any excess water and let the lentils cool.

2. In a large mixing bowl, combine the cooked lentils, diced cucumber, diced bell pepper, chopped red onion, halved cherry tomatoes, sliced Kalamata olives, crumbled feta cheese, and chopped fresh parsley.

3. In a small bowl, whisk together the extra virgin olive oil, red wine vinegar, dried oregano, salt, and pepper to make the dressing.

4. Pour the dressing over the lentil mixture in the large bowl and toss everything together until evenly coated.

5. Taste and adjust the seasoning, adding more salt and pepper if needed.

6. Serve the Mediterranean lentil salad chilled or at room temperature as a delicious and nutritious side dish or light meal.

7. Enjoy your flavorful and refreshing Mediterranean lentil salad!

52. Roasted Vegetable Pasta Salad

Ingredients:
- 8 ounces pasta (such as penne or fusilli)
- 2 cups mixed vegetables (bell peppers, zucchini, cherry tomatoes, etc.), chopped
- 2 tablespoons olive oil
- Salt and pepper to taste
- 1/4 cup basil leaves, chopped
- 1/4 cup grated Parmesan cheese (optional)
- For the dressing:
  - 3 tablespoons extra virgin olive oil
  - 2 tablespoons balsamic vinegar
  - 1 teaspoon Dijon mustard
  - 1 clove garlic, minced
  - Salt and pepper to taste

Instructions:

1. Preheat your oven to 400°F (200°C). Line a baking sheet with parchment paper.

2. Toss the mixed vegetables with olive oil, salt, and pepper on the prepared baking sheet.

3. Roast the vegetables in the preheated oven for 20-25 minutes, or until tender and slightly caramelized, stirring halfway through cooking.

4. Meanwhile, cook the pasta according to the package instructions until al dente. Drain and rinse under cold water to stop the cooking process. Let it cool slightly.

5. In a small bowl, whisk together the extra virgin olive oil, balsamic vinegar, Dijon mustard, minced garlic, salt, and pepper to make the dressing.

6. In a large mixing bowl, combine the cooked pasta, roasted vegetables, chopped basil leaves, and grated Parmesan cheese (if using).

7. Pour the dressing over the pasta and vegetable mixture in the bowl, and toss everything together until evenly coated.

8. Taste and adjust the seasoning, adding more salt and pepper if needed.

9. Serve the roasted vegetable pasta salad chilled or at room temperature as a delicious and colorful side dish or light meal.

10. Enjoy your flavorful and satisfying roasted vegetable pasta salad!

53. Portobello Mushroom and Vegetable Fajitas

Ingredients:
- 4 large Portobello mushrooms, sliced
- 1 onion, sliced
- 1 bell pepper, sliced
- 1 zucchini, sliced
- 2 tablespoons olive oil
- 2 cloves garlic, minced
- 1 tablespoon chili powder
- 1 teaspoon ground cumin
- 1 teaspoon paprika
- Salt and pepper to taste
- Juice of 1 lime
- 8 small flour tortillas
- Optional toppings: salsa, guacamole, sour cream, shredded cheese, chopped cilantro

Instructions:

1. In a large skillet or grill pan, heat 1 tablespoon of olive oil over medium-high heat.

2. Add the sliced Portobello mushrooms to the skillet and cook for 5-7 minutes, stirring occasionally, until they start to soften and brown.

3. Add the sliced onion, bell pepper, and zucchini to the skillet with the mushrooms.

4. Drizzle the remaining tablespoon of olive oil over the vegetables, and sprinkle with minced garlic, chili powder, ground cumin, paprika, salt, and pepper. Stir to combine.

5. Cook the vegetable mixture for another 5-7 minutes, stirring occasionally, until the vegetables are tender but still slightly crisp.

6. Squeeze the lime juice over the vegetable mixture and stir to combine.

7. Warm the flour tortillas in a separate skillet or microwave according to the package instructions.

8. To serve, spoon the Portobello mushroom and vegetable mixture onto the warm tortillas.

9. Top with your favorite toppings such as salsa, guacamole, sour cream, shredded cheese, and chopped cilantro.

10. Roll up the tortillas and serve the Portobello mushroom and vegetable fajitas immediately. Enjoy your delicious and flavorful fajitas!

54. Baked Sweet Potato Fries

Ingredients:
- 2 large sweet potatoes
- 2 tablespoons olive oil
- 1 teaspoon garlic powder
- 1 teaspoon paprika
- 1/2 teaspoon cumin
- Salt and pepper to taste
- Optional: chopped fresh herbs (such as parsley or rosemary) for garnish

Instructions:

1. Preheat your oven to 425°F (220°C). Line a baking sheet with parchment paper or aluminum foil.

2. Wash and peel the sweet potatoes, then cut them into thin strips or wedges, about 1/4 inch thick.

3. In a large mixing bowl, toss the sweet potato strips with olive oil, garlic powder, paprika, cumin, salt, and pepper until evenly coated.

4. Arrange the seasoned sweet potato strips in a single layer on the prepared baking sheet, making sure they're not overlapping.

5. Bake the sweet potato fries in the preheated oven for 20-25 minutes, flipping halfway through, until they are golden brown and crispy on the outside and tender on the inside.

6. Once done, remove the sweet potato fries from the oven and let them cool slightly on the baking sheet.

7. Season with additional salt and pepper if desired, and garnish with chopped fresh herbs before serving.

8. Serve the baked sweet potato fries hot as a delicious and healthier snack or side dish.

9. Enjoy your crispy and flavorful sweet potato fries!

These baked sweet potato fries are easy to make and packed with flavor. They're perfect for snacking, serving as a side dish, or enjoying with your favorite dipping sauce.

55. Kale and Quinoa Salad with Avocado

Ingredients:
- 1 cup quinoa, rinsed
- 2 cups water or vegetable broth
- 4 cups kale, stems removed and chopped
- 1 ripe avocado, diced
- 1/4 cup dried cranberries or raisins
- 1/4 cup chopped almonds or walnuts, toasted
- 2 tablespoons lemon juice
- 2 tablespoons extra virgin olive oil
- 1 clove garlic, minced
- Salt and pepper to taste

Instructions:
1. In a medium saucepan, bring the water or vegetable broth to a boil. Add the rinsed quinoa, reduce heat to low, cover, and simmer for 15-20 minutes, or until the quinoa is cooked and the liquid is absorbed. Remove from heat and let it cool slightly.

2. In a large mixing bowl, massage the chopped kale with a little olive oil for a few minutes to help soften it.

3. Add the cooked quinoa, diced avocado, dried cranberries or raisins, and toasted chopped almonds or walnuts to the bowl with the kale.

4. In a small bowl, whisk together the lemon juice, extra virgin olive oil, minced garlic, salt, and pepper to make the dressing.

5. Pour the dressing over the kale and quinoa mixture in the large bowl and toss everything together until evenly coated.

6. Taste and adjust the seasoning, adding more salt and pepper if needed.

7. Serve the kale and quinoa salad with avocado chilled or at room temperature as a delicious and nutritious side dish or light meal.

8. Enjoy your flavorful and satisfying kale and quinoa salad with avocado!

This salad is packed with healthy ingredients and vibrant flavors, making it a perfect option for lunch or dinner.

56. Roasted Vegetable and Hummus Wraps

Ingredients:
- 1 cup mixed vegetables (such as bell peppers, zucchini, red onion, cherry tomatoes), chopped
- 1 tablespoon olive oil
- Salt and pepper to taste
- 4 large tortillas or wraps
- 1 cup hummus
- Fresh spinach leaves or lettuce for topping
- Optional: crumbled feta cheese, sliced avocado, chopped fresh herbs (such as parsley or cilantro)

Instructions:

1. Preheat your oven to 400°F (200°C). Line a baking sheet with parchment paper.

2. Toss the chopped mixed vegetables with olive oil, salt, and pepper on the prepared baking sheet.

3. Roast the vegetables in the preheated oven for 20-25 minutes, or until tender and slightly caramelized, stirring halfway through cooking.

4. Warm the tortillas or wraps according to the package instructions, if desired.

5. Spread a generous layer of hummus onto each tortilla or wrap.

6. Arrange a handful of fresh spinach leaves or lettuce on top of the hummus.

7. Once the roasted vegetables are done, spoon them onto the tortillas or wraps on top of the spinach leaves.

8. If using, sprinkle crumbled feta cheese, sliced avocado, and chopped fresh herbs over the roasted vegetables.

9. Roll up the tortillas or wraps tightly, enclosing the filling.

10. Slice the wraps in half diagonally, if desired, and serve immediately.

11. Enjoy your delicious and satisfying roasted vegetable and hummus wraps!

These wraps are versatile and can be customized with your favorite vegetables and toppings. They're perfect for a quick and nutritious lunch or dinner option.

57. Vegetarian Chili with Sweet Potatoes

Ingredients:
- 2 tablespoons olive oil
- 1 onion, diced
- 2 cloves garlic, minced
- 2 sweet potatoes, peeled and diced
- 1 bell pepper, diced
- 1 zucchini, diced
- 1 can (15 ounces) black beans, drained and rinsed
- 1 can (15 ounces) kidney beans, drained and rinsed
- 1 can (15 ounces) diced tomatoes
- 2 cups vegetable broth
- 2 tablespoons tomato paste
- 2 teaspoons chili powder
- 1 teaspoon ground cumin
- 1 teaspoon smoked paprika
- Salt and pepper to taste
- Optional toppings: chopped cilantro, sliced avocado, shredded cheese, sour cream, lime wedges

Instructions:

1. In a large pot or Dutch oven, heat the olive oil over medium heat.

2. Add the diced onion and minced garlic to the pot, and sauté for 2-3 minutes until softened and fragrant.

3. Add the diced sweet potatoes, bell pepper, and zucchini to the pot, and cook for another 5 minutes, stirring occasionally.

4. Stir in the drained and rinsed black beans and kidney beans, diced tomatoes (with their juices), vegetable broth, tomato paste, chili powder, ground cumin, smoked paprika, salt, and pepper.

5. Bring the chili to a boil, then reduce the heat to low and let it simmer, partially covered, for 20-25 minutes, or until the sweet potatoes are tender and the chili has thickened slightly.

6. Taste and adjust the seasoning, adding more salt and pepper if needed.

7. Serve the vegetarian chili hot, garnished with chopped cilantro, sliced avocado, shredded cheese, sour cream, and lime wedges if desired. Enjoy your delicious and comforting vegetarian chili with sweet potatoes!

58. Grilled Vegetable Skewers with Chimichurri Sauce

Ingredients:
- For the vegetable skewers:
  - 2 zucchinis, sliced into rounds
  - 1 red bell pepper, cut into chunks
  - 1 yellow bell pepper, cut into chunks
  - 1 red onion, cut into chunks
  - 8-10 cherry tomatoes
  - Wooden or metal skewers, soaked if using wooden ones

- *For the chimichurri sauce:*
  - 1 cup fresh parsley leaves, chopped
  - 1/4 cup fresh cilantro leaves, chopped
  - 3 cloves garlic, minced
  - 1 shallot, minced
  - 1/4 cup red wine vinegar
  - 1/2 cup extra virgin olive oil
  - 1 teaspoon dried oregano
  - 1/2 teaspoon red pepper flakes (adjust to taste)
  - Salt and pepper to taste

Instructions:

1. Preheat your grill to medium-high heat.

2. Thread the sliced zucchinis, bell pepper chunks, onion chunks, and cherry tomatoes onto the skewers, alternating the vegetables as desired.

3. In a small bowl, combine all the ingredients for the chimichurri sauce: chopped parsley, chopped cilantro, minced garlic, minced shallot, red wine vinegar, extra virgin olive oil, dried oregano, red pepper flakes, salt, and pepper. Stir well to combine.

4. Brush the vegetable skewers with a little olive oil to prevent sticking.

5. Place the vegetable skewers on the preheated grill and cook for 8-10 minutes, turning occasionally, until the vegetables are tender and lightly charred.

6. Once the vegetable skewers are done, remove them from the grill and transfer them to a serving platter.

7. Drizzle the chimichurri sauce over the grilled vegetable skewers or serve it on the side for dipping.

8. Serve the grilled vegetable skewers with chimichurri sauce hot as a delicious and colorful appetizer or side dish. Enjoy the flavorful combination of grilled vegetables with the zesty chimichurri sauce!

These grilled vegetable skewers with chimichurri sauce are perfect for summer cookouts, barbecues, or any time you want to enjoy a tasty and healthy dish.

59. Lentil and Vegetable Stuffed Tomatoes

Ingredients:
- 1 teaspoon dried oregano
- 1/2 teaspoon dried thyme
- Salt and pepper to taste
- 1/4 cup breadcrumbs (optional)
- Fresh parsley or basil for garnish
- 4 large tomatoes
- 1 cup cooked lentils
- 1 cup mixed vegetables (such as bell peppers, zucchini, carrots), finely diced
- 1/2 onion, finely chopped
- 2 tablespoons olive oil
- 2 cloves garlic, minced

Instructions:

1. Preheat your oven to 375°F (190°C).

2. Cut the tops off the tomatoes and scoop out the seeds and pulp from the centers using a spoon, leaving a hollow shell. Set aside.

3. In a large skillet, heat olive oil over medium heat. Add the chopped onion and minced garlic, and sauté until softened and fragrant, about 2-3 minutes.

4. Add the diced mixed vegetables to the skillet and cook for another 5-7 minutes, or until they are tender.

5. Stir in the cooked lentils, dried oregano, dried thyme, salt, and pepper. Cook for an additional 2-3 minutes to allow the flavors to meld together.

6. Remove the skillet from heat and let the lentil and vegetable mixture cool slightly.

7. Stuff each hollowed-out tomato with the lentil and vegetable mixture, pressing it down gently to pack it in.

8. If desired, sprinkle breadcrumbs over the tops of the stuffed tomatoes for a crispy topping.

9. Place the stuffed tomatoes in a baking dish or on a baking sheet lined with parchment paper.

10. Bake in the preheated oven for 20-25 minutes, or until the tomatoes are tender and the filling is heated through.

11. Once done, remove the stuffed tomatoes from the oven and let them cool for a few minutes before serving.

12. Garnish with fresh parsley or basil before serving. Enjoy your delicious and nutritious lentil and vegetable stuffed tomatoes as a satisfying vegetarian meal or side dish!

60. Roasted Brussels Sprouts and Apple Salad

Ingredients:
- 1 lb Brussels sprouts, trimmed and halved
- 2 tablespoons olive oil
- Salt and pepper to taste
- 1 large apple, thinly sliced
- 1/4 cup dried cranberries or raisins
- 1/4 cup chopped pecans or walnuts, toasted
- 2 tablespoons balsamic vinegar
- 1 tablespoon honey or maple syrup
- 2 tablespoons extra virgin olive oil
- 1 teaspoon Dijon mustard
- Salt and pepper to taste
- Optional: crumbled goat cheese or feta cheese for topping

Instructions:

1. Preheat your oven to 400°F (200°C). Line a baking sheet with parchment paper.

2. In a large bowl, toss the halved Brussels sprouts with olive oil, salt, and pepper until evenly coated.

3. Spread the Brussels sprouts out in a single layer on the prepared baking sheet.

4. Roast the Brussels sprouts in the preheated oven for 20-25 minutes, or until they are tender and caramelized, stirring halfway through cooking.

5. While the Brussels sprouts are roasting, prepare the dressing. In a small bowl, whisk together the balsamic vinegar, honey or maple syrup, extra virgin olive oil, Dijon mustard, salt, and pepper until well combined.

6. Once the Brussels sprouts are done roasting, transfer them to a large mixing bowl.

7. Add the thinly sliced apple, dried cranberries or raisins, and chopped toasted pecans or walnuts to the bowl with the roasted Brussels sprouts.

8. Drizzle the dressing over the salad and toss everything together until evenly coated.

9. Taste and adjust the seasoning, adding more salt and pepper if needed.

10. If desired, sprinkle crumbled goat cheese or feta cheese over the top of the salad before serving.

11. Serve the roasted Brussels sprouts and apple salad warm or at room temperature as a delicious and nutritious side dish or light meal. Enjoy your flavorful and satisfying salad!

This roasted Brussels sprouts and apple salad is perfect for fall and winter gatherings, and it's packed with delicious flavors and textures that everyone will love.

61. Vegetable Stir-Fry with Brown Rice

Ingredients:
- 2 cups cooked brown rice
- 2 tablespoons vegetable oil
- 2 cloves garlic, minced
- 1 tablespoon ginger, minced
- 1 onion, sliced
- 2 carrots, julienned
- 1 bell pepper, sliced
- 1 cup broccoli florets
- 1 cup snap peas or snow peas
- 1 cup mushrooms, sliced
- 1/4 cup soy sauce (or tamari for gluten-free option)
- 2 tablespoons oyster sauce (optional, omit for vegan option)
- 1 tablespoon sesame oil
- 1 tablespoon rice vinegar
- 1 tablespoon honey or maple syrup (optional, for sweetness)
- Salt and pepper to taste
- Optional garnishes: sliced green onions, sesame seeds

Instructions:

1. In a small bowl, whisk together soy sauce, oyster sauce (if using), sesame oil, rice vinegar, honey or maple syrup (if using), and a pinch of salt and pepper. Set aside.

2. Heat vegetable oil in a large skillet or wok over medium-high heat. Add minced garlic and ginger, and stir-fry for 1-2 minutes until fragrant.

3. Add sliced onion and julienned carrots to the skillet. Stir-fry for 2-3 minutes until slightly softened.

4. Add sliced bell pepper, broccoli florets, snap peas or snow peas, and sliced mushrooms to the skillet. Stir-fry for an additional 3-4 minutes until the vegetables are tender-crisp.

5. Pour the prepared sauce over the vegetables in the skillet. Stir well to coat all the vegetables in the sauce.

6. Cook for another 1-2 minutes until the sauce has thickened slightly and the vegetables are evenly coated.

7. Taste and adjust the seasoning, adding more salt and pepper if needed. Serve the vegetable stir-fry over cooked brown rice.

8. Garnish with sliced green onions and sesame seeds, if desired. Enjoy your delicious and nutritious vegetable stir-fry with brown rice!

This vegetable stir-fry is packed with colorful and nutritious veggies, and it's a quick and easy meal that's perfect for busy weeknights. Feel free to customize the vegetables and sauce according to your preferences!

62. Mediterranean Chickpea and Vegetable Salad

Ingredients:
- 1 can (15 ounces) chickpeas (garbanzo beans), drained and rinsed
- 1 cucumber, diced
- 1 bell pepper (red, yellow, or orange), diced
- 1 cup cherry tomatoes, halved
- 1/4 cup red onion, thinly sliced
- 1/4 cup Kalamata olives, pitted and sliced
- 1/4 cup crumbled feta cheese
- 1/4 cup chopped fresh parsley
- For the dressing:
  - 2 tablespoons extra virgin olive oil
  - 1 tablespoon lemon juice
  - 1 clove garlic, minced
  - 1 teaspoon dried oregano
  - Salt and pepper to taste

Instructions:
1. In a large mixing bowl, combine the chickpeas, diced cucumber, diced bell pepper, halved cherry tomatoes, thinly sliced red onion, sliced Kalamata olives, crumbled feta cheese, and chopped fresh parsley.

2. In a small bowl, whisk together the extra virgin olive oil, lemon juice, minced garlic, dried oregano, salt, and pepper to make the dressing.

3. Pour the dressing over the chickpea and vegetable mixture in the large bowl.

4. Toss everything together until evenly coated with the dressing.

5. Taste and adjust the seasoning, adding more salt and pepper if needed.

6. Serve the Mediterranean chickpea and vegetable salad chilled or at room temperature as a delicious and nutritious side dish or light meal.

7. Enjoy your flavorful and refreshing salad!

This Mediterranean chickpea and vegetable salad is packed with protein, fiber, and flavor, making it a satisfying and healthy option for lunch or dinner. Feel free to customize the salad with your favorite Mediterranean ingredients and herbs!

63. Sweet Potato and Black Bean Veggie Burgers

Ingredients:
- 2 cups cooked black beans (or 1 can, drained and rinsed)
- 2 cups mashed sweet potatoes (about 2 medium sweet potatoes, cooked and mashed)
- 1/2 cup breadcrumbs (or oats for a gluten-free option)
- 1/4 cup finely chopped onion
- 2 cloves garlic, minced
- 1 teaspoon ground cumin
- 1 teaspoon chili powder
- 1/2 teaspoon smoked paprika
- Salt and pepper to taste
- 1 tablespoon olive oil (for cooking)
- Burger buns and toppings of choice (lettuce, tomato, avocado, etc.)

Instructions:

1. Preheat your oven to 375°F (190°C). Line a baking sheet with parchment paper.

2. In a large mixing bowl, combine the cooked black beans, mashed sweet potatoes, breadcrumbs, chopped onion, minced garlic, ground cumin, chili powder, smoked paprika, salt, and pepper.

3. Use a potato masher or fork to mash the mixture until well combined, but still slightly chunky.

4. Divide the mixture into equal portions and shape them into burger patties.

5. Place the patties on the prepared baking sheet and brush both sides lightly with olive oil.

6. Bake the veggie burgers in the preheated oven for 25-30 minutes, flipping halfway through cooking, until they are firm and lightly browned on the outside.

7. Once done, remove the veggie burgers from the oven and let them cool slightly before serving.

8. Serve the sweet potato and black bean veggie burgers on burger buns with your favorite toppings, such as lettuce, tomato, avocado, and condiments. Enjoy your delicious and satisfying veggie burgers!

These sweet potato and black bean veggie burgers are packed with flavor and nutrients, making them a perfect option for a meatless meal. They're also freezer-friendly, so you can make a batch ahead of time and enjoy them whenever you want!

64. Grilled Portobello Mushroom Tacos

Ingredients:
- 4 large Portobello mushrooms, stems removed
- 2 tablespoons olive oil
- 2 cloves garlic, minced
- 1 teaspoon ground cumin
- 1 teaspoon chili powder
- Salt and pepper to taste
- 8 small corn tortillas
- Toppings of choice: shredded lettuce, diced tomatoes, sliced avocado, chopped cilantro, lime wedges, salsa, etc.

Instructions:

1. Preheat your grill to medium-high heat.

2. In a small bowl, whisk together the olive oil, minced garlic, ground cumin, chili powder, salt, and pepper.

3. Brush both sides of the Portobello mushrooms with the seasoned olive oil mixture.

4. Place the mushrooms on the preheated grill and cook for 4-5 minutes per side, or until they are tender and grill marks appear.

5. Once done, remove the grilled Portobello mushrooms from the grill and let them cool slightly.

6. Slice the grilled Portobello mushrooms into thin strips.

7. Warm the corn tortillas on the grill or in a skillet until they are soft and pliable.

8. To assemble the tacos, fill each warm tortilla with sliced grilled Portobello mushrooms and your desired toppings, such as shredded lettuce, diced tomatoes, sliced avocado, chopped cilantro, and a squeeze of lime juice.

9. Serve the grilled Portobello mushroom tacos immediately. Enjoy your delicious and flavorful tacos!

These grilled Portobello mushroom tacos are a delicious and satisfying vegetarian option for taco night. They're packed with savory flavors and hearty textures that will satisfy even meat lovers! Feel free to customize the toppings according to your preferences.

65. Roasted Garlic Cauliflower Mash

Ingredients:
- 1 head of cauliflower, cut into florets
- 4 cloves garlic, peeled
- 2 tablespoons olive oil
- Salt and pepper to taste
- 2 tablespoons butter or olive oil (for vegan option)
- 1/4 cup milk or vegetable broth (for vegan option)
- Optional: chopped fresh herbs (such as parsley or chives) for garnish

Instructions:

1. Preheat your oven to 400°F (200°C).

2. Place the cauliflower florets and peeled garlic cloves on a baking sheet lined with parchment paper.

3. Drizzle the cauliflower and garlic with olive oil, and season with salt and pepper to taste. Toss to coat evenly.

4. Roast in the preheated oven for 25-30 minutes, or until the cauliflower is tender and caramelized, and the garlic cloves are soft and golden brown.

5. Once roasted, transfer the cauliflower and garlic to a food processor or blender.

6. Add the butter or olive oil and milk or vegetable broth to the food processor or blender.

7. Blend until smooth and creamy, scraping down the sides as needed. If the mixture is too thick, you can add more milk or vegetable broth a little at a time until you reach your desired consistency.

8. Taste and adjust the seasoning, adding more salt and pepper if needed. Transfer the roasted garlic cauliflower mash to a serving dish.

9. Garnish with chopped fresh herbs, if desired, and serve hot. Enjoy your creamy and flavorful roasted garlic cauliflower mash as a delicious and nutritious side dish!

This roasted garlic cauliflower mash is a healthier alternative to traditional mashed potatoes and pairs well with a variety of main dishes. It's also gluten-free and can easily be made vegan by using olive oil and vegetable broth instead of butter and milk.

66. Veggie Stir-Fry with Quinoa

Ingredients:
- 1 cup quinoa, rinsed
- 2 cups water or vegetable broth
- 2 tablespoons vegetable oil
- 2 cloves garlic, minced
- 1 tablespoon ginger, minced
- 1 onion, thinly sliced
- 2 carrots, julienned
- 1 bell pepper, thinly sliced
- 1 cup broccoli florets
- 1 cup snap peas or snow peas
- 1 cup sliced mushrooms
- 1/4 cup soy sauce (or tamari for gluten-free option)
- 2 tablespoons hoisin sauce
- 1 tablespoon rice vinegar
- 1 tablespoon sesame oil
- Optional: sliced green onions and sesame seeds for garnish

Instructions:

1. In a medium saucepan, combine the rinsed quinoa and water or vegetable broth. Bring to a boil, then reduce the heat to low, cover, and simmer for 15-20 minutes, or until the quinoa is cooked and the liquid is absorbed. Remove from heat and let it sit, covered, for 5 minutes. Fluff with a fork and set aside.

2. In a large skillet or wok, heat vegetable oil over medium-high heat.

3. Add minced garlic and minced ginger to the skillet, and cook for 1-2 minutes until fragrant. Add thinly sliced onion to the skillet and cook for 2-3 minutes until softened.

4. Add julienned carrots, thinly sliced bell pepper, broccoli florets, snap peas or snow peas, and sliced mushrooms to the skillet. Stir-fry for 5-7 minutes until the vegetables are tender-crisp.

5. In a small bowl, whisk together soy sauce (or tamari), hoisin sauce, rice vinegar, and sesame oil to make the sauce.

6. Pour the sauce over the vegetables in the skillet and toss everything together until evenly coated.

7. Cook for another 1-2 minutes until the sauce has thickened slightly. Taste and adjust the seasoning, adding more soy sauce or salt if needed.

8. Serve the veggie stir-fry over cooked quinoa. Garnish with sliced green onions and sesame seeds, if desired. Enjoy your delicious and nutritious veggie stir-fry with quinoa!

This veggie stir-fry with quinoa is a healthy and satisfying meal that's packed with protein, fiber, and vitamins. It's perfect for a quick and easy dinner option that the whole family will love!

67. White Bean and Kale Soup

Ingredients:
- 2 tablespoons olive oil
- 1 onion, diced
- 2 carrots, diced
- 2 celery stalks, diced
- 3 cloves garlic, minced
- 1 teaspoon dried thyme
- 1 teaspoon dried rosemary
- 6 cups vegetable broth
- 2 cans (15 ounces each) white beans (such as cannellini beans or navy beans), drained and rinsed
- 1 bunch kale, stems removed and leaves chopped
- Salt and pepper to taste
- Optional toppings: grated Parmesan cheese, red pepper flakes, crusty bread

Instructions:

1. In a large pot or Dutch oven, heat olive oil over medium heat.

2. Add diced onion, carrots, and celery to the pot. Cook, stirring occasionally, for about 5-7 minutes until the vegetables are softened.

3. Add minced garlic, dried thyme, and dried rosemary to the pot. Cook for another 1-2 minutes until fragrant.

4. Pour vegetable broth into the pot and bring to a simmer.

5. Add drained and rinsed white beans to the pot. Simmer for about 10-15 minutes to allow the flavors to meld together.

6. Stir in chopped kale leaves and continue to simmer for an additional 5-7 minutes until the kale is wilted and tender.

7. Season the soup with salt and pepper to taste, adjusting as needed.

8. Once done, remove the soup from heat and let it cool slightly before serving.

9. Ladle the white bean and kale soup into bowls.

10. Optionally, garnish with grated Parmesan cheese and red pepper flakes. Serve with crusty bread if desired. Enjoy your comforting and nutritious white bean and kale soup!

This soup is packed with fiber, protein, and vitamins from the beans and kale, making it a healthy and satisfying meal option for lunch or dinner. Feel free to customize the soup with your favorite herbs and spices!

68. Roasted Beet and Feta Salad

Ingredients:
- 3-4 medium-sized beets, peeled and diced
- 2 tablespoons olive oil
- Salt and pepper to taste
- 4 cups mixed salad greens (such as spinach, arugula, or mixed baby greens)
- 1/2 cup crumbled feta cheese
- 1/4 cup chopped walnuts or pecans, toasted
- Balsamic glaze or vinaigrette dressing

Instructions:

1. Preheat your oven to 400°F (200°C).

2. Place the diced beets on a baking sheet lined with parchment paper.

3. Drizzle olive oil over the beets and season with salt and pepper to taste. Toss to coat evenly.

4. Roast the beets in the preheated oven for 25-30 minutes, or until they are tender and caramelized, stirring halfway through cooking.

5. Once roasted, remove the beets from the oven and let them cool slightly.

6. In a large mixing bowl, combine the mixed salad greens with the roasted beets.

7. Sprinkle crumbled feta cheese and chopped toasted walnuts or pecans over the top of the salad.

8. Drizzle balsamic glaze or vinaigrette dressing over the salad, to taste.

9. Toss everything together until evenly coated with the dressing.

10. Serve the roasted beet and feta salad immediately as a delicious and nutritious side dish or light meal.

11. Enjoy your flavorful and vibrant salad!

This roasted beet and feta salad is packed with color, flavor, and nutrients, making it a perfect option for a healthy and refreshing dish. Feel free to customize the salad with your favorite toppings anddressing!

69. Tofu Scramble with Veggies

Ingredients:
- 1 block (14-16 ounces) firm tofu, drained and pressed
- 2 tablespoons olive oil or neutral cooking oil
- 1 small onion, diced
- 2 cloves garlic, minced
- 1 bell pepper, diced
- 1 cup sliced mushrooms
- 2 cups fresh spinach or kale, chopped
- 2 tablespoons nutritional yeast (optional, for a cheesy flavor)
- 1 teaspoon ground turmeric
- Salt and pepper to taste
- Optional toppings: chopped green onions, diced tomatoes, sliced avocado, hot sauce

Instructions:

1. Heat olive oil in a large skillet over medium heat.

2. Add diced onion and minced garlic to the skillet. Sauté for 2-3 minutes until softened and fragrant.

3. Crumble the drained and pressed tofu into the skillet using your hands or a fork.

4. Cook the tofu, stirring occasionally, for about 5 minutes to allow it to brown slightly.

5. Add diced bell pepper and sliced mushrooms to the skillet. Cook for another 3-4 minutes until the vegetables are tender.

6. Stir in chopped spinach or kale, nutritional yeast (if using), ground turmeric, salt, and pepper. Cook for an additional 2-3 minutes until the greens are wilted.

7. Taste and adjust the seasoning, adding more salt and pepper if needed.

8. Once done, remove the tofu scramble from heat.

9. Serve the tofu scramble hot, garnished with chopped green onions, diced tomatoes, sliced avocado, and hot sauce if desired. Enjoy your delicious and protein-packed tofu scramble with veggies!

This tofu scramble with veggies is a versatile and satisfying dish that's perfect for breakfast, brunch, or any time of day. Feel free to customize it with your favorite vegetables and topping

70. Cauliflower Fried Rice with Edamame

Ingredients:
- 2 eggs, beaten (optional)
- 3 tablespoons soy sauce (or tamari for gluten-free option)
- 1 teaspoon Sriracha or chili sauce (optional)
- Salt and pepper to taste
- 2 green onions, chopped (for garnish)
- Sesame seeds (for garnish)
- 1 small head cauliflower, grated or finely chopped (or about 4 cups cauliflower rice)
- 2 tablespoons sesame oil or olive oil
- 2 cloves garlic, minced
- 1 tablespoon rice vinegar
- 1 small onion, diced
- 1 carrot, diced
- 1 bell pepper, diced
- 1 cup frozen edamame, thawed

Instructions:

1. If you haven't already, prepare the cauliflower rice by grating or finely chopping the cauliflower into rice-sized pieces.

2. Heat sesame oil or olive oil in a large skillet or wok over medium heat.

3. Add minced garlic and diced onion to the skillet. Sauté for 2-3 minutes until softened and fragrant.

4. Add diced carrot and bell pepper to the skillet. Cook for another 3-4 minutes until the vegetables are tender-crisp.

5. Stir in cauliflower rice and thawed edamame. Cook for 5-6 minutes, stirring occasionally, until the cauliflower is tender.

6. If using, push the cauliflower mixture to one side of the skillet and pour beaten eggs into the empty side. Allow the eggs to cook for a minute or two, then scramble them with a spatula until cooked through. Mix the scrambled eggs into the cauliflower mixture.

7. In a small bowl, whisk together soy sauce (or tamari), rice vinegar, and Sriracha or chili sauce (if using). Pour the sauce over the cauliflower mixture in the skillet.

8. Stir everything together until evenly coated with the sauce. Taste and adjust the seasoning, adding more salt and pepper if needed.

10. Once done, remove the cauliflower fried rice from heat. Serve hot, garnished with chopped green onions and sesame seeds. Enjoy your flavorful and nutritious cauliflower fried rice with edamame!

This cauliflower fried rice with edamame is a healthier alternative to traditional fried rice and is packed with protein and fiber. It's a delicious and satisfying meal that's perfect for a quick and easy dinner option. Feel free to customize it with your favorite vegetables and spices!

71. Roasted Brussels Sprouts and Butternut Squash

Ingredients:
- 1 lb Brussels sprouts, trimmed and halved
- 1 small butternut squash, peeled, seeded, and diced
- 2 tablespoons olive oil
- 2 cloves garlic, minced
- 1 teaspoon dried thyme
- Salt and pepper to taste
- Optional: balsamic glaze or maple syrup for drizzling

Instructions:

1. Preheat your oven to 400°F (200°C). Line a baking sheet with parchment paper.

2. In a large mixing bowl, combine the halved Brussels sprouts and diced butternut squash.

3. Drizzle olive oil over the vegetables and add minced garlic, dried thyme, salt, and pepper. Toss to coat evenly.

4. Spread the Brussels sprouts and butternut squash out in a single layer on the prepared baking sheet.

5. Roast in the preheated oven for 25-30 minutes, stirring halfway through cooking, until the vegetables are tender and caramelized.

6. Once done, remove the roasted Brussels sprouts and butternut squash from the oven.

7. If desired, drizzle with balsamic glaze or maple syrup for extra flavor.

8. Serve hot as a delicious and nutritious side dish or add to salads, grain bowls, or pasta dishes.

9. Enjoy your flavorful and colorful roasted Brussels sprouts and butternut squash!

This roasted Brussels sprouts and butternut squash dish is perfect for autumn and winter meals. It's packed with flavor and nutrients, making it a healthy and satisfying addition to any meal. Feel free to customize the seasoning and add your favorite herbs or spices!

72. Quinoa Stuffed Portobello Mushrooms

Ingredients:
- 4 large Portobello mushrooms, stems removed
- 1 cup quinoa, rinsed
- 2 cups vegetable broth or water
- 2 tablespoons olive oil
- 1 small onion, diced
- 2 cloves garlic, minced
- 1 bell pepper, diced
- 1 cup spinach, chopped
- 1/4 cup chopped fresh parsley or basil
- 1/4 cup grated Parmesan cheese (optional, omit for vegan option)
- Salt and pepper to taste

Instructions:

1. Preheat your oven to 375°F (190°C). Line a baking sheet with parchment paper.

2. Place the Portobello mushrooms on the prepared baking sheet, gill side up.

3. In a medium saucepan, bring vegetable broth or water to a boil. Add rinsed quinoa, reduce heat to low, cover, and simmer for 15-20 minutes, or until the quinoa is cooked and liquid is absorbed. Remove from heat and let it sit, covered, for 5 minutes. Fluff with a fork and set aside.

4. In a large skillet, heat olive oil over medium heat. Add diced onion and minced garlic to the skillet. Sauté for 2-3 minutes until softened and fragrant.

5. Add diced bell pepper to the skillet and cook for another 2-3 minutes until softened.

6. Stir in chopped spinach and cook for 1-2 minutes until wilted.

7. Add cooked quinoa to the skillet with the vegetables. Stir in chopped fresh parsley or basil. Season with salt and pepper to taste. Cook for another minute to allow flavors to meld together.

8. If using, stir in grated Parmesan cheese until melted and combined with the quinoa mixture.

9. Spoon the quinoa mixture into the gill side of each Portobello mushroom, pressing down gently to pack it in.

10. Bake in the preheated oven for 15-20 minutes, or until the mushrooms are tender and the filling is heated through.

11. Once done, remove the stuffed Portobello mushrooms from the oven. Serve hot as a delicious and satisfying main dish or hearty side dish. Enjoy your flavorful and nutritious quinoa stuffed Portobello mushrooms

73. Grilled Vegetable and Tofu Kebabs

Ingredients:
- 1 block (14-16 ounces) firm tofu, pressed and cubed
- 2 bell peppers, cut into chunks
- 1 zucchini, sliced into rounds
- 1 yellow squash, sliced into rounds
- 1 red onion, cut into chunks
- 8-10 cherry tomatoes

- For the marinade:
- 1/4 cup olive oil
- 2 tablespoons balsamic vinegar
- 2 cloves garlic, minced
- 1 teaspoon dried herbs (such as thyme, oregano, or rosemary)
- Salt and pepper to taste
- Wooden or metal skewers

Instructions:

1. If you're using wooden skewers, soak them in water for at least 30 minutes to prevent them from burning on the grill.

2. In a small bowl, whisk together the olive oil, balsamic vinegar, minced garlic, dried herbs, salt, and pepper to make the marinade.

3. Place the cubed tofu and prepared vegetables in a large mixing bowl.

4. Pour the marinade over the tofu and vegetables, tossing to coat evenly. Let them marinate for at least 30 minutes, or longer if time allows.

5. Preheat your grill to medium-high heat.

6. Thread the marinated tofu and vegetables onto skewers, alternating the ingredients as desired.

7. Place the assembled kebabs on the preheated grill and cook for 10-12 minutes, turning occasionally, until the vegetables are tender and slightly charred, and the tofu is heated through.

8. Once done, remove the grilled vegetable and tofu kebabs from the grill. Serve hot as a delicious and nutritious main dish or hearty side dish. Enjoy your flavorful and colorful grilled vegetable and tofu kebabs!

These grilled vegetable and tofu kebabs are packed with flavor and protein, making them a perfect option for vegetarian BBQs or summer gatherings. They're also versatile, so feel free to customize them with your favorite vegetables and herbs!

74. Baked Sweet Potato Wedges

Ingredients:
- 2 medium sweet potatoes, washed and dried
- 2 tablespoons olive oil
- 1 teaspoon paprika
- 1/2 teaspoon garlic powder
- 1/2 teaspoon onion powder
- 1/2 teaspoon dried thyme (optional)
- Salt and pepper to taste

Instructions:

1. Preheat your oven to 425°F (220°C). Line a baking sheet with parchment paper or aluminum foil.

2. Cut the sweet potatoes into wedges. You can leave the skin on for extra texture and nutrients, or peel them if you prefer.

3. In a large mixing bowl, toss the sweet potato wedges with olive oil until evenly coated.

4. In a small bowl, mix together paprika, garlic powder, onion powder, dried thyme (if using), salt, and pepper.

5. Sprinkle the seasoning mixture over the sweet potato wedges and toss to coat evenly.

6. Arrange the seasoned sweet potato wedges in a single layer on the prepared baking sheet.

7. Bake in the preheated oven for 20-25 minutes, flipping halfway through cooking, until the sweet potato wedges are tender and golden brown on the edges.

8. Once done, remove the baked sweet potato wedges from the oven.

9. Serve hot as a delicious and nutritious side dish or snack.

10. Enjoy your flavorful and crispy baked sweet potato wedges!

These baked sweet potato wedges are a healthier alternative to regular fries and are packed with vitamins and fiber. They're perfect for serving alongside burgers, sandwiches, or as a standalone snack with your favorite dipping sauce. Feel free to customize the seasoning with your favorite herbs and spices!

75. Kale Caesar Salad with Roasted Chickpeas

Ingredients:
- 1 bunch kale, stems removed and torn
- 1 cup cooked chickpeas, tossed with olive oil, salt, and pepper, then roasted until crispy
- Grated Parmesan cheese or nutritional yeast
- Optional: cherry tomatoes, cucumber, croutons

For the Caesar dressing:
- 1/4 cup mayonnaise or vegan mayo
- 2 tbsp grated Parmesan cheese or nutritional yeast
- 2 tbsp lemon juice
- 1 tbsp Dijon mustard
- 1 clove garlic, minced
- 2 anchovy fillets, minced (optional)
- Salt and pepper to taste
- Water (to thin the dressing)

Instructions:
1. Massage kale with a little olive oil.

2. Make Caesar dressing by whisking together mayo, Parmesan, lemon juice, Dijon mustard, garlic, anchovies (optional), salt, and pepper. Thin with water if needed.

3. Toss kale with roasted chickpeas and dressing.

4. Top with grated Parmesan cheese or nutritional yeast.

5. Optional: Add cherry tomatoes, cucumber, and croutons.

6. Serve and enjoy!

76. Roasted Vegetable and Lentil Salad

Ingredients:
- 1 cup dried lentils (green or brown), rinsed
- 3 cups water or vegetable broth
- 2 cups mixed vegetables (such as bell peppers, zucchini, cherry tomatoes, red onion)
- 2 tablespoons olive oil
- Salt and pepper to taste
- 2 cups mixed salad greens (such as spinach, arugula, or mixed baby greens)
- 1/4 cup crumbled feta cheese or diced avocado (optional)
- Balsamic vinaigrette dressing

Instructions:
1. Preheat your oven to 400°F (200°C).

2. In a medium saucepan, bring water or vegetable broth to a boil. Add rinsed lentils, reduce heat to low, cover, and simmer for 20-25 minutes, or until lentils are tender but still hold their shape. Drain any excess liquid and set aside.

3. While the lentils are cooking, prepare the mixed vegetables. Cut them into bite-sized pieces and place them on a baking sheet lined with parchment paper.

4. Drizzle the vegetables with olive oil and season with salt and pepper to taste. Toss to coat evenly.

5. Roast the vegetables in the preheated oven for 20-25 minutes, or until they are tender and lightly browned, stirring halfway through cooking.

6. Once the lentils and vegetables are cooked, let them cool slightly.

7. In a large mixing bowl, combine the cooked lentils, roasted vegetables, and mixed salad greens. If using, add crumbled feta cheese or diced avocado to the salad.

8. Drizzle with balsamic vinaigrette dressing and toss everything together until evenly coated. Taste and adjust the seasoning, adding more salt and pepper if needed.

9. Serve the roasted vegetable and lentil salad as a delicious and nutritious main dish or hearty side salad. Enjoy your flavorful and satisfying salad!

This roasted vegetable and lentil salad is packed with protein, fiber, and vitamins, making it a perfect option for a healthy and satisfying meal. Feel free to customize it with your favorite vegetables and toppings, and enjoy!

77. Black Bean and Sweet Potato Enchiladas

Ingredients:
- 1 tbsp olive oil
- 1 small onion, diced
- 2 cloves garlic, minced
- 1 tsp ground cumin
- 1 tsp chili powder
- 1/2 tsp smoked paprika
- 2 cups cooked black beans
- 1 large sweet potato, diced
- 1 cup corn kernels
- 1 cup enchilada sauce
- 8-10 corn tortillas
- 1 cup shredded cheese
- Salt and pepper to taste
- Optional toppings: cilantro, avocado, sour cream, jalapeños

Instructions:

1. Sauté onion and garlic in olive oil. Add spices, sweet potato, beans, and corn. Cook until tender.

2. Spread enchilada sauce in a baking dish. Fill tortillas with the mixture, roll, and place in the dish.

3. Pour remaining sauce over the enchiladas, sprinkle with cheese.

4. Bake at 375°F (190°C) for 20-25 mins.

5. Serve hot, garnished with optional toppings.

Enjoy your delicious black bean and sweet potato enchiladas!

78. Grilled Vegetable Fajita Bowls

Ingredients:
- 2 bell peppers, sliced
- 1 onion, sliced
- 1 zucchini, sliced
- 1 yellow squash, sliced
- 1 cup cherry tomatoes
- 2 tablespoons olive oil
- 1 tablespoon fajita seasoning (store-bought or homemade)
- Salt and pepper to taste
- 1 cup cooked rice or quinoa
- 1 cup black beans, drained and rinsed
- 1 avocado, sliced
- Fresh cilantro, chopped (for garnish)
- Lime wedges (for serving)
- Optional toppings: salsa, sour cream or Greek yogurt, shredded cheese, sliced jalapeños

Instructions:
1. Preheat your grill to medium-high heat.

2. In a large mixing bowl, toss the sliced bell peppers, onion, zucchini, yellow squash, and cherry tomatoes with olive oil and fajita seasoning until evenly coated. Season with salt and pepper to taste.

3. Place the seasoned vegetables in a grill basket or directly on the grill grates. Grill for 8-10 minutes, flipping occasionally, until the vegetables are tender and lightly charred.

4. While the vegetables are grilling, prepare the rice or quinoa according to package instructions.

5. Once the vegetables are done, assemble the fajita bowls. Divide the cooked rice or quinoa among serving bowls.

6. Top each bowl with grilled vegetables, black beans, sliced avocado, and any desired toppings.

7. Garnish with fresh chopped cilantro and serve with lime wedges on the side. Enjoy your delicious and colorful grilled vegetable fajita bowls!

These grilled vegetable fajita bowls are a satisfying and nutritious meal that's perfect for summer grilling or a quick weeknight dinner. Feel free to customize them with your favorite vegetables and toppings, and enjoy the vibrant flavors!

79. Mediterranean Lentil Soup

Ingredients:
- 1 tablespoon olive oil
- 1 onion, diced
- 2 carrots, diced
- 2 stalks celery, diced
- 3 cloves garlic, minced
- 1 teaspoon dried oregano
- 1 teaspoon dried thyme
- 1 teaspoon ground cumin
- 1 cup dried brown lentils, rinsed and drained
- 4 cups vegetable broth
- 1 (14.5-ounce) can diced tomatoes
- 2 cups spinach or kale, chopped
- Salt and pepper to taste
- Lemon wedges (for serving)
- Fresh parsley, chopped (for garnish)
- Optional toppings: crumbled feta cheese, Greek yogurt, toasted bread

Instructions:
1. Heat olive oil in a large pot over medium heat. Add diced onion, carrots, and celery. Cook for 5-6 minutes until vegetables are softened.

2. Add minced garlic, dried oregano, dried thyme, and ground cumin. Cook for 1-2 minutes until fragrant.

3. Stir in dried brown lentils, vegetable broth, and diced tomatoes (with their juices). Bring to a boil.

4. Reduce heat to low, cover, and simmer for 25-30 minutes, or until lentils are tender.

5. Stir in chopped spinach or kale and cook for an additional 5 minutes until wilted. Season with salt and pepper to taste.

6. Ladle the soup into bowls. Squeeze a lemon wedge over each bowl and garnish with chopped parsley.

7. Serve hot with optional toppings like crumbled feta cheese, Greek yogurt, or toasted bread. Enjoy your hearty and flavorful Mediterranean lentil soup!

This Mediterranean lentil soup is packed with protein, fiber, and vibrant Mediterranean flavors. It's a comforting and nutritious meal that's perfect for chilly days or anytime you're craving a warm and satisfying bowl of soup. Feel free to customize it with your favorite herbs and spices!

80. Roasted Vegetable and Quinoa Salad

Ingredients:
- 1 cup quinoa, rinsed
- 2 cups vegetable broth or water
- 2 cups mixed vegetables (e.g., bell peppers, zucchini, cherry tomatoes, red onion), chopped
- 2 tablespoons olive oil
- Salt and pepper to taste
- 1 teaspoon dried oregano
- 1 teaspoon dried thyme
- 1/4 cup crumbled feta cheese or diced avocado (optional)
- 2 cups mixed greens (e.g., spinach, arugula, or mixed baby greens)
- Balsamic vinaigrette dressing

Instructions:
1. Preheat your oven to 400°F (200°C). Line a baking sheet with parchment paper.

2. In a medium saucepan, bring vegetable broth or water to a boil. Add quinoa, reduce heat to low, cover, and simmer for 15-20 minutes, or until quinoa is cooked and liquid is absorbed. Fluff with a fork and set aside to cool.

3. While the quinoa is cooking, place the chopped mixed vegetables on the prepared baking sheet. Drizzle with olive oil, and season with salt, pepper, dried oregano, and dried thyme. Toss to coat evenly.

4. Roast the vegetables in the preheated oven for 20-25 minutes, stirring halfway through, until they are tender and lightly browned.

5. In a large mixing bowl, combine the cooked quinoa, roasted vegetables, and mixed greens. Toss to combine.

6. If using, add crumbled feta cheese or diced avocado. Drizzle with balsamic vinaigrette dressing and toss until everything is evenly coated.

7. Serve the roasted vegetable and quinoa salad warm or at room temperature. Enjoy your delicious and nutritious salad!

This roasted vegetable and quinoa salad is a flavorful and healthy meal, perfect for lunch or dinner. Customize it with your favorite vegetables and toppings for a versatile dish that's packed with nutrients.

81. Portobello Mushroom Veggie Burgers

Ingredients:
- 4 large Portobello mushrooms, stems removed and gills scraped out
- 2 tablespoons olive oil
- 1 tablespoon balsamic vinegar
- 1 teaspoon soy sauce or tamari (for gluten-free option)
- 1/2 teaspoon garlic powder
- 1/2 teaspoon onion powder
- Salt and pepper to taste
- 4 whole wheat or gluten-free burger buns
- Toppings: lettuce, tomato, avocado, red onion, pickles, mustard, ketchup, or your favorite burger toppings

Instructions:
1. Preheat your grill or grill pan to medium-high heat.

2. In a small bowl, whisk together olive oil, balsamic vinegar, soy sauce or tamari, garlic powder, onion powder, salt, and pepper.

3. Brush the marinade on both sides of each Portobello mushroom cap.

4. Place the mushrooms on the grill, gill side down, and cook for 5-7 minutes. Flip and cook for another 5-7 minutes, or until the mushrooms are tender and have nice grill marks.

5. Toast the burger buns on the grill for 1-2 minutes, if desired.

6. Assemble the burgers by placing a grilled Portobello mushroom on the bottom half of each bun. Add your desired toppings and the top half of the bun.

7. Serve immediately and enjoy your flavorful Portobello mushroom veggie burgers!

These Portobello mushroom veggie burgers are a hearty and delicious alternative to traditional beef burgers. They're easy to make, packed with umami flavor, and can be customized with your favorite toppings. Perfect for a summer BBQ or a weeknight dinner!

82. Garlic Roasted Brussels Sprouts

Ingredients:
- 1 pound Brussels sprouts, trimmed and halved
- 3 tablespoons olive oil
- 4 cloves garlic, minced
- Salt and pepper to taste
- 1 tablespoon balsamic vinegar (optional)
- 1/4 cup grated Parmesan cheese (optional)

Instructions:
1. Preheat your oven to 400°F (200°C). Line a baking sheet with parchment paper or lightly grease it.

2. In a large bowl, toss the halved Brussels sprouts with olive oil, minced garlic, salt, and pepper until evenly coated.

3. Spread the Brussels sprouts in a single layer on the prepared baking sheet.

4. Roast in the preheated oven for 20-25 minutes, stirring halfway through, until the Brussels sprouts are tender and golden brown on the edges.

5. If using, drizzle with balsamic vinegar and sprinkle with Parmesan cheese during the last 5 minutes of roasting.

6. Remove from the oven and transfer to a serving dish.

7. Serve hot and enjoy your garlic roasted Brussels sprouts!

These garlic roasted Brussels sprouts are a simple and delicious side dish, perfect for any meal. The optional balsamic vinegar and Parmesan cheese add extra flavor and richness.

83. Quinoa and Edamame Salad

Ingredients:
- 1 cup quinoa, rinsed
- 2 cups water or vegetable broth
- 1 cup shelled edamame (fresh or frozen)
- 1 cup cherry tomatoes, halved
- 1 cucumber, diced
- 1/4 cup red onion, finely diced
- 1/4 cup fresh parsley or cilantro, chopped
- 2 tablespoons olive oil
- 2 tablespoons lemon juice
- 1 tablespoon rice vinegar
- Salt and pepper to taste

Instructions:

1. In a medium saucepan, bring water or vegetable broth to a boil. Add the quinoa, reduce heat to low, cover, and simmer for 15-20 minutes, or until the quinoa is cooked and the liquid is absorbed. Fluff with a fork and set aside to cool.

2. While the quinoa is cooking, prepare the edamame according to package instructions (usually boiling for 3-5 minutes) and then drain and cool.

3. In a large mixing bowl, combine the cooked quinoa, edamame, cherry tomatoes, cucumber, red onion, and parsley or cilantro.

4. In a small bowl, whisk together the olive oil, lemon juice, rice vinegar, salt, and pepper.

5. Pour the dressing over the quinoa and vegetable mixture and toss until everything is well coated.

6. Taste and adjust seasoning as needed.

7. Serve chilled or at room temperature.

Enjoy your refreshing and nutritious quinoa and edamame salad! This salad is perfect as a light lunch, a side dish, or a potluck contribution.

84. Roasted Vegetable Grain Bowls

Ingredients:
- 1 cup quinoa, farro, or brown rice
- 2 cups vegetable broth or water
- 2 cups mixed vegetables (e.g., bell peppers, zucchini, cherry tomatoes, carrots), chopped
- 2 tablespoons olive oil
- 1 teaspoon dried oregano
- 1 teaspoon dried thyme
- Salt and pepper to taste
- 1 cup chickpeas, drained and rinsed
- 1 avocado, sliced
- 1/4 cup feta cheese or diced avocado (optional)
- Fresh herbs (e.g., parsley, cilantro, basil) for garnish
- Balsamic vinaigrette or tahini dressing

Instructions:

1. Preheat your oven to 400°F (200°C). Line a baking sheet with parchment paper.

2. Cook the grain (quinoa, farro, or brown rice) according to package instructions using vegetable broth or water. Set aside to cool.

3. While the grain is cooking, place the chopped mixed vegetables on the prepared baking sheet. Drizzle with olive oil, and season with dried oregano, dried thyme, salt, and pepper. Toss to coat evenly.

4. Roast the vegetables in the preheated oven for 20-25 minutes, stirring halfway through, until they are tender and lightly browned.

5. In a large mixing bowl, combine the cooked grain, roasted vegetables, and chickpeas.

6. Divide the mixture into serving bowls. Top with sliced avocado, feta cheese (if using), and fresh herbs.

7. Drizzle with balsamic vinaigrette or tahini dressing. Serve warm or at room temperature.

Enjoy your delicious and nutritious roasted vegetable grain bowls! These bowls are versatile and can be customized with your favorite grains, vegetables, and toppings.

85. Lentil Sloppy Joes with Sweet Potato Buns

Ingredients:
For Lentil Sloppy Joes:
- 1 cup lentils
- 1 onion, diced
- 2 cloves garlic, minced
- 1 bell pepper, diced
- 1 can (14 oz) crushed tomatoes
- 2 tablespoons tomato paste
- 1 tablespoon maple syrup
- 1 tablespoon soy sauce
- 1 teaspoon chili powder
- Salt and pepper to taste

For Sweet Potato Buns:
- 2 large sweet potatoes
- Olive oil
- Salt and pepper to taste

Instructions:

1. Cook lentils according to package instructions until tender.

2. In a separate pan, sauté onion, garlic, and bell pepper until softened.

3. Add cooked lentils, crushed tomatoes, tomato paste, maple syrup, soy sauce, and chili powder to the pan. Stir to combine.

4. Simmer the mixture for about 10 minutes, allowing flavors to meld. Season with salt and pepper to taste.

5. While the lentil mixture is simmering, preheat the oven to 400°F (200°C).

6. Slice sweet potatoes into rounds, about 1/2 inch thick.

7. Place sweet potato rounds on a baking sheet, drizzle with olive oil, and season with salt and pepper.

8. Bake sweet potato rounds for 20-25 minutes, or until tender and slightly caramelized. Serve lentil sloppy joe mixture on top of sweet potato buns.

86. Grilled Portobello Mushroom Sandwiches

Ingredients:
- 4 large portobello mushrooms
- 4 tablespoons balsamic vinegar
- 2 tablespoons olive oil
- 2 cloves garlic, minced
- Salt and pepper to taste
- 4 slices of your favorite bread
- Optional toppings: lettuce, tomato, avocado, cheese

Instructions:
1. Preheat your grill to medium-high heat.

2. Clean the portobello mushrooms and remove the stems.

3. In a small bowl, whisk together the balsamic vinegar, olive oil, minced garlic, salt, and pepper.

4. Brush the marinade over both sides of the portobello mushrooms.

5. Place the mushrooms on the grill, gill side down, and cook for about 4-5 minutes per side, or until tender and grill marks form.

6. While the mushrooms are grilling, toast the slices of bread.

7. Once the mushrooms are cooked, assemble the sandwiches by placing the grilled portobello mushrooms on the toasted bread slices.

8. Add any desired toppings such as lettuce, tomato, avocado, or cheese.

9. Serve immediately and enjoy your Grilled Portobello Mushroom Sandwiches!

87. Baked Tofu and Broccoli Stir-Fry

Ingredients:
- 1 block (14 oz) extra firm tofu, pressed and cubed
- 1 head of broccoli, cut into florets
- 2 tablespoons soy sauce
- 2 tablespoons hoisin sauce
- 1 tablespoon sesame oil
- 2 cloves garlic, minced
- 1 teaspoon ginger, minced
- Salt and pepper to taste
- Cooked rice, for serving

Instructions:

1. Preheat your oven to 400°F (200°C).

2. Place the cubed tofu on a baking sheet lined with parchment paper or lightly greased.

3. Bake the tofu for 25-30 minutes, flipping halfway through, until golden and crispy.

4. While the tofu is baking, steam the broccoli florets until tender, about 5-7 minutes.

5. In a small bowl, whisk together the soy sauce, hoisin sauce, sesame oil, minced garlic, and minced ginger.

6. Once the tofu is baked and broccoli is steamed, heat a large skillet over medium heat.

7. Add the baked tofu and steamed broccoli to the skillet, then pour the sauce over them.

8. Stir-fry for a few minutes until everything is well coated and heated through.

9. Season with salt and pepper to taste.

10. Serve the baked tofu and broccoli stir-fry over cooked rice.

11. Enjoy your delicious and nutritious meal!

88. Cauliflower Rice Veggie Burrito Bowls

Ingredients:
For Cauliflower Rice:
- 1 head of cauliflower, grated or pulsed into rice-like consistency
- 1 tablespoon olive oil
- Salt and pepper to taste

For Veggie Burrito Bowls:
- 1 can (15 oz) black beans, drained and rinsed
- 1 bell pepper, diced
- 1 cup corn kernels (fresh, canned, or frozen)
- 1 avocado, sliced
- 1 tomato, diced
- 1/4 cup chopped fresh cilantro
- Juice of 1 lime
- Optional toppings: shredded cheese, sour cream, salsa

Instructions:
1. Prepare the cauliflower rice by grating or pulsing the cauliflower florets in a food processor until they resemble rice grains.

2. Heat olive oil in a large skillet over medium heat. Add the cauliflower rice and cook for 5-7 minutes, stirring occasionally, until it's tender.

3. Season the cauliflower rice with salt and pepper to taste, then remove it from the heat and set aside.

4. In the same skillet, add the black beans, diced bell pepper, and corn kernels. Cook for 5-7 minutes, or until the vegetables are tender.

5. Once the vegetables are cooked, assemble the burrito bowls by dividing the cauliflower rice among serving bowls.

6. Top the cauliflower rice with the black bean and vegetable mixture.

7. Add sliced avocado, diced tomato, and chopped cilantro on top of each bowl.

8. Squeeze fresh lime juice over the burrito bowls for extra flavor.

9. Serve with optional toppings like shredded cheese, sour cream, or salsa. Enjoy your Cauliflower Rice Veggie Burrito Bowls!

89. White Bean and Vegetable Soup

Ingredients:
- 2 tablespoons olive oil
- 1 onion, diced
- 2 carrots, diced
- 2 celery stalks, diced
- 3 cloves garlic, minced
- 4 cups vegetable broth
- 2 cans (15 oz each) white beans, drained and rinsed
- 1 can (14.5 oz) diced tomatoes
- 1 teaspoon dried thyme
- 1 teaspoon dried oregano
- Salt and pepper to taste
- Fresh parsley, chopped, for garnish (optional)

Instructions:

1. Heat olive oil in a large pot over medium heat.

2. Add diced onion, carrots, and celery to the pot. Cook, stirring occasionally, until the vegetables are softened, about 5-7 minutes.

3. Add minced garlic to the pot and cook for another minute until fragrant.

4. Pour in vegetable broth, white beans, diced tomatoes (with their juices), dried thyme, and dried oregano. Stir to combine.

5. Bring the soup to a boil, then reduce the heat to low. Let it simmer uncovered for about 15-20 minutes to allow the flavors to meld together.

6. Season the soup with salt and pepper to taste.

7. If desired, use an immersion blender to partially blend the soup for a creamier texture, leaving some chunks of vegetables and beans intact.

8. Serve the soup hot, garnished with chopped fresh parsley if desired.

9. Enjoy your hearty and comforting White Bean and Vegetable Soup!

90. Roasted Beet and Goat Cheese Salad

Ingredients:
- 3 medium beets, peeled and cubed
- 2 tablespoons olive oil
- Salt and pepper to taste
- 4 cups mixed salad greens
- 1/4 cup crumbled goat cheese
- 1/4 cup chopped walnuts (optional)
- Balsamic vinaigrette dressing

Instructions:
1. Preheat your oven to 400°F (200°C).

2. Place the cubed beets on a baking sheet lined with parchment paper.

3. Drizzle olive oil over the beets and toss to coat evenly. Season with salt and pepper.

4. Roast the beets in the preheated oven for 25-30 minutes, or until tender and slightly caramelized, stirring halfway through.

5. While the beets are roasting, prepare your salad greens in a large bowl.

6. Once the beets are done roasting, let them cool slightly before adding them to the salad greens.

7. Sprinkle crumbled goat cheese and chopped walnuts (if using) over the salad.

8. Drizzle balsamic vinaigrette dressing over the salad, tossing gently to combine.

9. Serve immediately and enjoy your flavorful Roasted Beet and Goat Cheese Salad!

91. Tofu Veggie Scramble with Sweet Potato Hash

Ingredients:

For Tofu Veggie Scramble:
- 1 block (14 oz) firm tofu, drained and crumbled
- 1 tablespoon olive oil
- 1 small onion, diced
- 1 bell pepper, diced
- 1 cup sliced mushrooms
- 2 cups spinach leaves
- 2 cloves garlic, minced
- 1 teaspoon turmeric
- Salt and pepper to taste

For Sweet Potato Hash:
- 2 medium sweet potatoes, peeled and diced
- 2 tablespoons olive oil
- 1 teaspoon paprika
- Salt and pepper to taste

Instructions:

For Tofu Veggie Scramble:

1. Heat olive oil in a large skillet over medium heat.

2. Add diced onion, bell pepper, and sliced mushrooms to the skillet. Cook until softened, about 5-7 minutes.

3. Add minced garlic to the skillet and cook for another minute until fragrant.

4. Add crumbled tofu to the skillet, along with turmeric, salt, and pepper. Stir well to combine.

5. Cook the tofu mixture for 5-7 minutes, stirring occasionally, until heated through and slightly browned.

6. Add spinach leaves to the skillet and cook until wilted, about 2-3 minutes. Remove the skillet from heat and set aside.

For Sweet Potato Hash:

1. Heat olive oil in a separate skillet over medium heat.

2. Add diced sweet potatoes to the skillet and cook until tender and slightly crispy, about 10-12 minutes, stirring occasionally.

3. Season the sweet potatoes with paprika, salt, and pepper, stirring to coat evenly.

Divide the tofu veggie scramble and sweet potato hash among serving plates. Serve hot and enjoy your delicious Tofu Veggie Scramble with Sweet Potato Hash!

92. Vegetable Stir-Fry with Brown Rice Noodles

Ingredients:
For Vegetable Stir-Fry:
- 2 tablespoons sesame oil
- 2 cloves garlic, minced
- 1 small onion, sliced

For Brown Rice Noodles:
- 8 oz brown rice noodles
- 1 bell pepper, sliced
- 1 carrot, julienned
- 1 cup broccoli florets
- 1 cup snow peas, trimmed
- 1 cup sliced mushrooms
- 1 cup bean sprouts
- 2 tablespoons soy sauce
- 1 tablespoon hoisin sauce (optional)
- Salt and pepper to taste
- Crushed red pepper flakes (optional, for heat)

Instructions:

1. Cook the brown rice noodles according to the package instructions. Once cooked, drain and set aside.

2. Heat sesame oil in a large skillet or wok over medium-high heat.

3. Add minced garlic and sliced onion to the skillet. Stir-fry for 1-2 minutes until fragrant.

4. Add sliced bell pepper, julienned carrot, broccoli florets, snow peas, and sliced mushrooms to the skillet. Stir-fry for 5-7 minutes until the vegetables are tender-crisp.

5. Add bean sprouts to the skillet and stir-fry for another 1-2 minutes.

6. In a small bowl, mix together soy sauce and hoisin sauce (if using). Pour the sauce over the vegetable stir-fry and toss to coat evenly.

7. Season with salt, pepper, and crushed red pepper flakes (if using) to taste.

8. Add the cooked brown rice noodles to the skillet and toss everything together until well combined and heated through.

9. Remove from heat and serve hot.

10. Enjoy your flavorful Vegetable Stir-Fry with Brown Rice Noodles!

93. Roasted Brussels Sprouts and Pomegranate Salad

Ingredients:
- 1 lb Brussels sprouts, trimmed and halved
- 2 tablespoons olive oil
- Salt and pepper to taste
- 1/2 cup pomegranate arils
- 1/4 cup chopped pecans (optional)
- 2 tablespoons balsamic glaze or reduction
- 2 cups mixed salad greens

Instructions:
1. Preheat your oven to 400°F (200°C).

2. Toss the halved Brussels sprouts with olive oil, salt, and pepper on a baking sheet until evenly coated.

3. Roast the Brussels sprouts in the preheated oven for 20-25 minutes, or until tender and caramelized, stirring halfway through.

4. While the Brussels sprouts are roasting, prepare the salad greens in a large bowl.

5. Once the Brussels sprouts are done, let them cool slightly before adding them to the salad greens.

6. Sprinkle pomegranate arils and chopped pecans (if using) over the salad.

7. Drizzle balsamic glaze or reduction over the salad for extra flavor.

8. Toss everything gently to combine.

9. Serve immediately and enjoy your delicious Roasted Brussels Sprouts and Pomegranate Salad!

94. Quinoa Stuffed Bell Peppers

Ingredients:
- 4 large bell peppers, any color
- 1 cup quinoa, rinsed
- 2 cups vegetable broth or water
- 1 tablespoon olive oil
- 1 small onion, diced
- 2 cloves garlic, minced
- 1 zucchini, diced
- 1 carrot, diced
- 1 cup diced tomatoes (fresh or canned)
- 1 teaspoon dried oregano
- 1 teaspoon dried basil
- Salt and pepper to taste
- 1/2 cup shredded cheese (optional)

Instructions:

1. Preheat your oven to 375°F (190°C).

2. Cut the tops off the bell peppers and remove the seeds and membranes. Set aside.

3. In a medium saucepan, combine quinoa and vegetable broth or water. Bring to a boil, then reduce heat to low, cover, and simmer for 15-20 minutes, or until the quinoa is cooked and the liquid is absorbed.

4. In a large skillet, heat olive oil over medium heat. Add diced onion and minced garlic, and cook until softened and fragrant, about 2-3 minutes.

5. Add diced carrot and zucchini to the skillet, and cook for another 5 minutes until slightly tender.

6. Stir in diced tomatoes, dried oregano, dried basil, cooked quinoa, salt, and pepper. Cook for an additional 2-3 minutes to allow the flavors to meld.

7. Stuff each bell pepper with the quinoa and vegetable mixture, pressing down gently to pack it in.

8. Place the stuffed bell peppers in a baking dish, standing upright.

9. If using cheese, sprinkle shredded cheese over the tops of the stuffed peppers.

10. Cover the baking dish with aluminum foil and bake in the preheated oven for 25-30 minutes, or until the bell peppers are tender.

11. Remove the foil during the last 5 minutes of baking to allow the cheese to melt and lightly brown. Serve hot and enjoy your delicious Quinoa Stuffed Bell Peppers!

95. Grilled Vegetable and Halloumi Skewers

Ingredients:
- 1 block (8 oz) halloumi cheese, cut into cubes
- 1 zucchini, sliced into rounds
- 1 bell pepper, cut into chunks
- 1 red onion, cut into chunks
- 8-10 cherry tomatoes
- 2 tablespoons olive oil
- 2 cloves garlic, minced
- Juice of 1 lemon
- 1 teaspoon dried oregano
- Salt and pepper to taste
- Wooden skewers, soaked in water for at least 30 minutes

Instructions:
1. Preheat your grill to medium-high heat.

2. In a small bowl, whisk together olive oil, minced garlic, lemon juice, dried oregano, salt, and pepper to make the marinade.

3. Thread the halloumi cheese cubes, zucchini slices, bell pepper chunks, red onion chunks, and cherry tomatoes onto the soaked wooden skewers, alternating between the vegetables and cheese.

4. Brush the vegetable and halloumi skewers with the marinade, coating them evenly.

5. Place the skewers on the preheated grill and cook for 8-10 minutes, turning occasionally, until the vegetables are tender and the halloumi is lightly charred.

6. Remove the skewers from the grill and serve hot.

7. Enjoy your flavorful Grilled Vegetable and Halloumi Skewers as a delicious appetizer or main course!

96. Baked Sweet Potato Falafels

Ingredients:
- 2 medium sweet potatoes, peeled and cubed
- 1 can (15 oz) chickpeas, drained and rinsed
- 2 cloves garlic, minced
- 2 tablespoons olive oil
- 2 tablespoons tahini
- 1 tablespoon lemon juice
- 1 teaspoon ground cumin
- 1 teaspoon ground coriander
- 1/2 teaspoon smoked paprika
- Salt and pepper to taste
- 1/4 cup chopped fresh parsley
- 1/4 cup chickpea flour or all-purpose flour
- Olive oil spray or cooking spray

Instructions:

1. Preheat your oven to 375°F (190°C).

2. Place the cubed sweet potatoes in a microwave-safe bowl and microwave on high for 5-6 minutes, or until they are tender.

3. In a food processor, combine the cooked sweet potatoes, chickpeas, minced garlic, olive oil, tahini, lemon juice, ground cumin, ground coriander, smoked paprika, salt, and pepper. Blend until smooth.

4. Transfer the mixture to a mixing bowl and stir in the chopped fresh parsley and chickpea flour (or all-purpose flour) until well combined. The mixture should be thick enough to form into balls.

5. Shape the mixture into small falafel balls, about 1-2 tablespoons each, and place them on a baking sheet lined with parchment paper.

6. Lightly spray the falafels with olive oil spray or cooking spray.

7. Bake in the preheated oven for 25-30 minutes, or until the falafels are golden brown and crispy on the outside.

8. Remove from the oven and let them cool slightly before serving.

9. Serve the baked sweet potato falafels with your favorite dipping sauce or in pita bread with salad and tahini sauce.

10. Enjoy your delicious and nutritious Baked Sweet Potato Falafels!

97. Kale and White Bean Salad

Ingredients:
- 1 bunch kale, stems removed and leaves chopped
- 1 can (15 oz) white beans, such as cannellini beans, drained and rinsed
- 1/4 cup diced red onion
- 1/4 cup chopped fresh parsley
- 1/4 cup grated Parmesan cheese (optional)
- 2 tablespoons olive oil
- 2 tablespoons lemon juice
- 1 teaspoon Dijon mustard
- Salt and pepper to taste

Instructions:

1. In a large mixing bowl, combine the chopped kale, white beans, diced red onion, and chopped fresh parsley.

2. In a small bowl, whisk together the olive oil, lemon juice, Dijon mustard, salt, and pepper to make the dressing.

3. Pour the dressing over the kale and white bean mixture. Toss until everything is well coated in the dressing.

4. If using, sprinkle grated Parmesan cheese over the salad and toss again to distribute evenly.

5. Let the salad sit for about 10-15 minutes to allow the flavors to meld together and the kale to slightly wilt.

6. Taste and adjust seasoning if needed, adding more salt, pepper, or lemon juice as desired.

7. Serve your Kale and White Bean Salad as a nutritious and flavorful side dish or light meal.

8. Enjoy!

98. Roasted Vegetable Grain Buddha Bowls

Ingredients:

For Roasted Vegetables:
- 2 cups mixed vegetables (such as carrots, bell peppers, zucchini, and cauliflower), chopped
- 2 tablespoons olive oil
- Salt and pepper to taste
- Optional: 1 teaspoon dried herbs (such as thyme or rosemary)

For Grain Base:
- 2 cups cooked grains (such as quinoa, brown rice, or farro)

For Assembly:
- 1 cup cooked chickpeas (canned or cooked from dry)
- 2 cups mixed salad greens
- 1 avocado, sliced
- 1/4 cup hummus
- Lemon wedges, for serving
- Optional toppings: toasted nuts or seeds, crumbled feta cheese, chopped fresh herbs

Instructions:

1. Preheat your oven to 400°F (200°C).

2. In a large mixing bowl, toss the chopped mixed vegetables with olive oil, salt, pepper, and dried herbs (if using) until evenly coated.

3. Spread the vegetables out on a baking sheet lined with parchment paper.

4. Roast the vegetables in the preheated oven for 20-25 minutes, or until they are tender and lightly caramelized, stirring halfway through.

5. While the vegetables are roasting, prepare your grain base by cooking your chosen grains according to package instructions.

6. Once the vegetables are done roasting and the grains are cooked, assemble your Buddha bowls.

7. Divide the cooked grains among serving bowls.

8. Top each bowl with a portion of the roasted vegetables, cooked chickpeas, mixed salad greens, and sliced avocado.

9. Add a dollop of hummus to each bowl. Sprinkle with any optional toppings you like, such as toasted nuts or seeds, crumbled feta cheese, or chopped fresh herbs.

11. Serve the Buddha bowls with lemon wedges on the side for squeezing over the top. Enjoy your nourishing and flavorful Roasted Vegetable Grain Buddha Bowls!

99. Sweet Potato and Black Bean Quesadillas

Ingredients:
- 2 medium sweet potatoes, peeled and diced
- 1 can (15 oz) black beans, drained and rinsed
- 1 cup shredded cheese (such as cheddar or Mexican blend)
- 4 large flour tortillas
- 1 tablespoon olive oil
- 1 teaspoon ground cumin
- 1 teaspoon chili powder
- Salt and pepper to taste
- Optional toppings: salsa, sour cream, avocado slices, chopped cilantro

Instructions:

1. Place the diced sweet potatoes in a microwave-safe bowl and microwave on high for 5-6 minutes, or until they are tender. Alternatively, you can steam or boil them until tender.

2. In a separate bowl, mash the cooked sweet potatoes with a fork until smooth.

3. Add the drained black beans, ground cumin, chili powder, salt, and pepper to the mashed sweet potatoes. Stir to combine.

4. Heat a large skillet over medium heat and lightly brush one side of each tortilla with olive oil.

5. Place one tortilla, oiled side down, in the skillet. Spread a layer of the sweet potato and black bean mixture evenly over the tortilla.

6. Sprinkle shredded cheese over the sweet potato and black bean mixture.

7. Place another tortilla on top, pressing down gently to adhere.

8. Cook the quesadilla for 3-4 minutes on each side, or until golden brown and crispy, and the cheese is melted.

9. Repeat the process with the remaining tortillas and filling.

10. Once cooked, remove the quesadillas from the skillet and let them cool slightly before slicing into wedges.

11. Serve the Sweet Potato and Black Bean Quesadillas with your favorite toppings such as salsa, sour cream, avocado slices, or chopped cilantro. Enjoy your delicious and satisfying quesadillas!

100. Mediterranean Grilled Vegetable Wraps

Ingredients:
For Grilled Vegetables:
- Zucchini, yellow squash, red bell pepper, red onion
- Olive oil, salt, pepper
- Optional: dried herbs

For Assembly:
- Whole wheat or spinach tortillas
- Hummus
- Mixed salad greens
- Feta cheese
- Kalamata olives
- Lemon wedges
- Optional: Tzatziki sauce or Greek yogurt

Instructions:
1. Grill sliced vegetables until tender.

2. Chop grilled vegetables into bite-sized pieces.

3. Warm tortillas and spread with hummus.

4. Layer with salad greens, grilled vegetables, feta, and olives.

5. Squeeze lemon juice, roll up tightly.

6. Serve with lemon wedges and optional dipping sauce.

7. Enjoy your Mediterranean Grilled Vegetable Wraps!

101. Lentil and Vegetable Pot Pies

Ingredients:
For Lentil and Vegetable Filling:
- 1 cup lentils
- 2 cups vegetable broth
- 2 tablespoons olive oil

For Pot Pie Crust:
- 1 package store-bought puff pastry or pie crust
- 1 onion, diced
- 2 carrots, diced
- 2 celery stalks, diced
- 2 cloves garlic, minced
- 1 teaspoon dried thyme
- 1 teaspoon dried rosemary
- Salt and pepper to taste
- 1 cup frozen peas
- 1/4 cup chopped fresh parsley

Instructions:

1. Preheat your oven to 375°F (190°C).

2. Rinse lentils and place them in a pot with vegetable broth. Bring to a boil, then reduce heat and simmer for 20-25 minutes, or until lentils are tender.

3. In a separate skillet, heat olive oil over medium heat. Add diced onion, carrots, and celery. Cook until softened, about 5-7 minutes.

4. Add minced garlic, dried thyme, and dried rosemary to the skillet. Cook for another minute until fragrant.

5. Stir cooked lentils (drained if necessary) into the skillet with the vegetables. Season with salt and pepper to taste.

6. Add frozen peas and chopped fresh parsley to the skillet. Stir to combine.

7. Roll out the store-bought puff pastry or pie crust and cut into circles large enough to cover individual ramekins or a baking dish.

8. Divide the lentil and vegetable filling among the ramekins or spread it evenly in the baking dish.

9. Cover each ramekin with a circle of puff pastry or pie crust.

10. Bake in the preheated oven for 20-25 minutes, or until the crust is golden brown and the filling is bubbly.

11. Let cool slightly before serving. Enjoy your comforting Lentil and Vegetable Pot Pies!

102. Roasted Garlic Cauliflower Steaks

Ingredients:
- 1 large head cauliflower
- 4 cloves garlic, minced
- 3 tablespoons olive oil
- 1 teaspoon paprika
- Salt and pepper to taste
- Optional garnish: chopped parsley, lemon wedges

Instructions:
1. Preheat your oven to 400°F (200°C).

2. Remove the leaves from the cauliflower head and trim the stem end, leaving the core intact.

3. Place the cauliflower head on a cutting board and slice it into 1-inch thick "steaks," cutting from top to bottom.

4. In a small bowl, mix together minced garlic, olive oil, paprika, salt, and pepper.

5. Brush both sides of each cauliflower steak with the garlic and oil mixture.

6. Place the cauliflower steaks on a baking sheet lined with parchment paper.

7. Roast in the preheated oven for 20-25 minutes, flipping halfway through, or until the cauliflower is tender and golden brown.

8. Remove from the oven and garnish with chopped parsley and lemon wedges if desired.

9. Serve hot and enjoy your flavorful Roasted Garlic Cauliflower Steaks!

103. Veggie Fried Cauliflower Rice

Ingredients:
- 1 head cauliflower
- 2 tablespoons sesame oil
- 1 onion, diced
- 2 carrots, diced
- 1 bell pepper, diced
- 2 cloves garlic, minced
- 1 cup frozen peas
- 2 eggs, beaten (optional)
- 3 tablespoons soy sauce
- 1 tablespoon rice vinegar
- 1 teaspoon grated ginger
- Salt and pepper to taste
- Green onions, chopped, for garnish

Instructions:
1. Wash and dry the cauliflower. Remove the leaves and cut the cauliflower into florets.

2. Working in batches, pulse the cauliflower florets in a food processor until they resemble rice grains.

3. Heat sesame oil in a large skillet or wok over medium heat.

4. Add diced onion, carrots, and bell pepper to the skillet. Stir-fry for 3-4 minutes until slightly softened.

5. Add minced garlic to the skillet and cook for another minute until fragrant.

6. Stir in the cauliflower rice and frozen peas. Cook for 5-6 minutes, stirring occasionally, until the cauliflower is tender.

7. Push the cauliflower rice mixture to one side of the skillet. Pour beaten eggs into the other side of the skillet and scramble until cooked through.

8. Once the eggs are cooked, mix them into the cauliflower rice mixture.

9. In a small bowl, whisk together soy sauce, rice vinegar, and grated ginger. Pour the sauce over the cauliflower rice and stir to combine.

10. Season with salt and pepper to taste. Garnish with chopped green onions before serving. Serve hot and enjoy your delicious Veggie Fried Cauliflower Rice!

104. Quinoa Tabbouleh Salad

Ingredients:
- 1 cup quinoa
- 2 cups water or vegetable broth
- 1 cup chopped cucumber
- 1 cup cherry tomatoes, halved
- 1/2 cup chopped fresh parsley
- 1/4 cup chopped fresh mint
- 1/4 cup chopped red onion
- 2 tablespoons olive oil
- 2 tablespoons lemon juice
- 1 clove garlic, minced
- Salt and pepper to taste

Instructions:

1. Rinse the quinoa under cold water using a fine mesh sieve.

2. In a medium saucepan, bring the water or vegetable broth to a boil. Add the rinsed quinoa, reduce the heat to low, cover, and simmer for 15-20 minutes, or until the quinoa is cooked and the liquid is absorbed.

3. Remove the cooked quinoa from the heat and let it cool to room temperature.

4. In a large mixing bowl, combine the cooled quinoa, chopped cucumber, halved cherry tomatoes, chopped fresh parsley, chopped fresh mint, and chopped red onion.

5. In a small bowl, whisk together the olive oil, lemon juice, minced garlic, salt, and pepper to make the dressing.

6. Pour the dressing over the quinoa tabbouleh salad and toss until everything is well coated.

7. Taste and adjust seasoning if needed.

8. Serve the quinoa tabbouleh salad chilled or at room temperature.

9. Enjoy your refreshing and nutritious Quinoa Tabbouleh Salad!

105. Grilled Portobellos with Roasted Veggies

Ingredients:
For Grilled Portobellos:
- 4 large portobello mushrooms, stems removed
- 2 tablespoons balsamic vinegar
- 2 tablespoons olive oil
- 2 cloves garlic, minced
- Salt and pepper to taste

For Roasted Veggies:
- 2 bell peppers, sliced
- 1 zucchini, sliced
- 1 yellow squash, sliced
- 1 red onion, sliced
- 2 tablespoons olive oil
- Salt and pepper to taste
- Optional: dried herbs like thyme or rosemary

Instructions:
1. Preheat your grill to medium-high heat.

2. In a small bowl, whisk together balsamic vinegar, olive oil, minced garlic, salt, and pepper.

3. Brush both sides of the portobello mushrooms with the balsamic mixture.

4. Place the mushrooms on the grill and cook for about 4-5 minutes per side, or until tender.
5. While the portobellos are grilling, preheat your oven to 400°F (200°C).

6. In a large mixing bowl, toss the sliced bell peppers, zucchini, yellow squash, and red onion with olive oil, salt, pepper, and optional dried herbs.

7. Spread the seasoned veggies out on a baking sheet lined with parchment paper.

8. Roast the vegetables in the preheated oven for 20-25 minutes, or until they are tender and slightly caramelized, stirring halfway through.

9. Once the portobellos and roasted veggies are done, serve them together on a platter.

10. Enjoy your delicious Grilled Portobellos with Roasted Veggies as a nutritious and flavorful meal!

*As we reach the end of **"Plant-Based Fatty Liver Diet Cookbook: Nourishing Your Liver, One Plant-Based Meal at a Time,"** I hope you feel empowered and inspired to take charge of your liver health through the power of plant-based nutrition. You've embarked on a journey that not only supports your liver but also enhances your overall well-being.*

This cookbook is more than just a collection of recipes; it's a guide to a healthier lifestyle. By choosing nutrient-rich, plant-based foods, you are making a profound commitment to your health. The recipes within these pages have been carefully crafted to provide you with delicious, satisfying meals that nourish your body and support your liver's function.

Remember, the path to better liver health is a journey, not a sprint. Small, consistent changes can lead to significant improvements over time. As you continue to explore and enjoy these plant-based meals, you'll find that healthy eating can be both enjoyable and sustainable.

I encourage you to keep experimenting with the recipes, trying new ingredients, and making this way of eating your own. Share your favorite dishes with family and friends, and inspire those around you to embrace the benefits of a plant-based diet.

Thank you for joining me on this journey toward better liver health. Your dedication to nourishing your body with wholesome, plant-based foods is a powerful step toward a healthier, happier future. Keep cooking, keep exploring, and keep nourishing your liver, one plant-based meal at a time.

Wishing you health and wellness,